The Health of the Nation

Averting the demise of universal healthcare

Edmund Stubbs (ed.)

Sally Al-Zaidy

John Ashton

Paul Corrigan

Stephen Dorrell

Phil Hammond

David J. Hunter

Steve Melton

Richard Murray

Mark Porter

Melanie Reid

Richard B. Saltman

Marco Viceconti

CIVITAS

First Published May 2016

© Civitas 2016
55 Tufton Street
London SW1P 3QL

email: books@civitas.org.uk

ISBN 978-1-906837-78-5

Independence: Civitas: Institute for the Study of Civil Society is a registered educational charity (No. 1085494) and a company limited by guarantee (No. 04023541). Civitas is financed from a variety of private sources to avoid over-reliance on any single or small group of donors.

Designed and typeset by
lukejefford.com

Printed in Great Britain by
4edge Limited, Essex

The Health of the Nation

Contents

Authors

Sally Al-Zaidy is the head of health policy at the BMA, where she has worked on a wide range of topics including commissioning, equity and rationing, integrated care and health service reform. In 2012 Sally graduated from the London School of Economics and Political Science with a distinction and the Brian Abel Smith Prize for outstanding performance in MSc Health Policy, Economics and Management.

John Ashton is the President of the Faculty of Public Health (FPH) for a term of three years (2013-2016). In this role John chairs the Board, Executive Committee and Fellowship Committee and represents FPH on a number of related bodies. John was North West Regional Director of Public Health and Regional Medical Officer from 1993 to 2006 and Director of Public Health and County Medical Officer for Cumbria from 2006 to 2013. Born in Liverpool in 1947, he was educated at Quarry Bank High School in Liverpool, the University of Newcastle-upon-Tyne Medical School and the London School of Hygiene and Tropical Medicine. He specialised in psychiatry, general practice, family planning and reproductive medicine before entering public health in 1976.

Paul Corrigan has had four careers. He was a social scientist specialising in inner city policy and practice.

He then worked as a senior manager in London local government. He has worked for the Labour party as education policy officer and was a special adviser to two secretaries of state for health and Tony Blair when he was prime minister. Since 2007 he has worked in the NHS and is now a management consultant and an executive coach.

Stephen Dorrell is a Senior Adviser to KPMG supporting the Global Health and Public Sector practices. In 2015 he was appointed Chair of the NHS Confederation. He was a Member of the UK Parliament from 1979-2015, serving as Secretary of State for Health 1995-97 and was Chair of the House of Commons Health Select Committee 2010-14. From 2005 to 2010 he was Co-Chair of the Conservative Policy Group on Public Service Improvement established by David Cameron to develop Conservative policy for public service reform. From 2008 to 2010 he was also a member of the cross party Commission on Public Service Reform convened by the Royal Society of Arts.

Phil Hammond is an NHS doctor working in chronic fatigue, an investigative journalist for Private Eye, a broadcaster for BBC Radio Bristol and the author of *Staying Alive - How to Get the Best from the NHS*. He is also a comedian, performing two shows at the 2016 Edinburgh Fringe: 'Life and Death (But Mainly Death)' and 'Dr Phil's NHS Revolution'.

David J. Hunter is Professor of Health Policy and Management at Durham University and Director of the Centre for Public Policy and Health. He is a non-executive director, NICE, and a special advisor to WHO Regional Office for Europe on health systems.

Steve Melton is Chief Executive of Circle Health, an employee co-owned company that runs hospitals and healthcare in the UK. He has been Chief Executive since 2013, and joined Circle after several decades in retail and manufacturing.

Richard Murray joined The King's Fund as Director of Policy in January 2014. He initially trained as an economist and spent five years in academia before joining the Department of Health as an economic adviser. Following this he spent a period of four years as a healthcare specialist at McKinsey & Co. In 2003 he returned to the Department of Health where he undertook a number of roles including Senior Economic Adviser, Director of Strategy, Director of Financial Planning and Chief Analyst, and finally Director of Finance, Quality, Strategy and Analysis. In 2013 he moved to NHS England as Chief Analyst before leaving to join The King's Fund.

Mark Porter is the leader of the British Medical Association as the elected BMA council chair. He is also an NHS consultant anaesthetist at University Hospitals Coventry and Warwickshire NHS Trust. He was appointed as Honorary Colonel of 202 (Midlands) Field Hospital, Royal Army Medical Corps in 2014 and holds a diploma in public administration from the University of Warwick.

Melanie Reid is a writer and columnist at The Times. In 2010 she fell off her horse and broke her neck. She started writing Spinal Column in The Times Magazine during her year-long stay in hospital and now, a tetraplegic, records the unvarnished realities of life for the chronically ill. She was UK Columnist of the Year in 2011 and in 2014 won the Edgar Wallace Award for Journalism and an Editorial Intelligence Comment Award. She is a graduate of Edinburgh University and has an honorary degree from Stirling University.

Richard B. Saltman is Professor of Health Policy and Management at the Emory University School of Public Health in Atlanta, Georgia. He was a co-founder of the European Observatory on Health Systems and Policies in Brussels in 1998, and is currently Associate Director of Research Policy and head of the Atlanta hub. He is an Adjunct Professor of Political Science at Emory University, a Visiting Professor at the London School of Economics and Political Science, and Visiting Professor at the Braun School of Public Health at the Hebrew University in Jerusalem.

Edmund Stubbs is Healthcare Researcher at Civitas. Edmund studied Biomedical Science at the University of Sheffield and health policy at the London School of Economics and Political Science. Edmund also worked as a healthcare assistant for four years at Addenbrooke's Hospital, Cambridge. His recent publications include 'Supplying the Demand for Nurses' and 'The Road to Healthcare Devolution'.

Marco Viceconti is Chair of Biomechanics at the Department of Mechanical Engineering and Professor Associate at the Department of Oncology and Metabolism at the University of Sheffield. He is currently serving as Executive Director of the Insigneo Institute of in silico medicine, a joint initiative between the University of Sheffield and the Sheffield Teaching Hospital NHS Foundation Trust.

Introduction

Edmund Stubbs

Evidence of a health system in demise appears in the media every day. Patients endure excessive waits for diagnosis and treatment and care pathways can be so fragmented that patients are often lost in the system. Many new drugs are becoming too expensive for prescription within the NHS's budget. Trusts have collectively overspent their budgets by more than £2 billion this year and clinical commissioning groups have to ration treatment in an effort to save money, even, as was recently the case in Devon, imposing controversial qualifying conditions for treatment such as the adoption of a healthier lifestyle. Britain's neglected mental health services cause some patients to travel long distances, or wait excessively long times with detrimental and sometimes fatal consequences. Repeated crises in accident and emergency (A&E) have become familiar headlines throughout recent winters with dramatic photographs and television footage of ambulances queuing outside emergency departments becoming commonplace. This is caused, in part, by patients remaining on wards for long periods after being declared medically fit to leave. Social isolation and a failing social care system mean that it is unsafe to discharge them. Community and primary health services fare no better, general practitioners warn of an impending crisis in the services they deliver, with appointment times currently too short to give to each patient the attention they need. Nurses and visiting social care workers on home visits similarly warn that they have insufficient time to meet the needs of their elderly patients, who are frequently socially isolated. In effect, the care sector in general appears to be failing.

NHS staff shortages are also a growing problem. To fill vacancies, nurses and doctors are necessarily recruited from overseas or are contracted from expensive specialist agencies. Staff morale is seemingly at an all-time low, so much so that the Health Secretary, Jeremy Hunt, has been spurred to commission a review of doctors' morale, the low level of which is reported to be an underlying cause of the recent failed contract negotiations. General practitioners add to the gloom, warning that not enough replacements are coming through the training system.

The NHS organisation is commonly accused of inefficiency, both in providing services and in procuring the material it needs to do so. Even efforts at improvement are sometimes said to erode service quality. For example, the NHS 111 phone line, staffed by handlers using spreadsheets and pro-formas to respond to enquiries rather than by clinically trained professionals has become a source of much recent public dissatisfaction.

So, what has brought Britain's health and care services to this precarious state? The principle factor seems to be the health of the nation. As fertility rates drop, and as the 'baby-boom' generation of the late 1940s and early 1950s reaches old age, it has resulted in a larger proportion of elderly people in relation to the rest of the population than was the case previously. Such elderly citizens generally require far more healthcare than do younger people. Britain's national healthcare system, in tandem with spectacular medical advances, has, in effect, kept many who would have previously died alive. Formerly short-term fatal diseases have now become chronic ones, requiring long-term, and therefore costly, treatment. In a 1942 report, William Beveridge, founder of Britain's welfare state, aimed to challenge what he termed the 'giants of too little', namely want, disease, idleness, ignorance and squalor. Such 'giants' have been replaced in contemporary affluent societies by Sir Julian Le Grand's 'giants of too much', the result of increasingly unhealthy diets, high in fats and sugars, and ever more sedentary lifestyles. In such modern societies, although life expectancy continues to rise, healthy life expectancy, that is years enjoying full health without moderate or severe disability, is increasing far more slowly.

Globally, many nations have striven to establish and maintain universal healthcare (UHC) for their citizens. A nation achieves UHC when its entire population is protected from the considerable costs that treating illness often involves, and ideally, offers equal access to healthcare services to all citizens regardless of wealth, geographical location, social class or ethnicity. At its foundation in 1948, Britain's National Health Service was a trailblazer, offering free-at-the-point-of-delivery healthcare according to need, rather than ability to pay, to all citizens. Today, 68 years later, almost every high-income nation, as well as some transitional economies, have some form of UHC. Unfortunately, it is becoming evident that meeting the high demand for expensive, modern healthcare is becoming prohibitive for many countries, including Britain, and that as a consequence such countries' UHC values are threatened. The situation is becoming serious. Now, as Paul Corrigan writes in his contribution to this publication: 'The NHS needs critical friends, not fawning adulation.' This book is a collection of the views of such 'critical friends' and attempts to support all those, professional or lay, of all parties and none, who wish to avert the demise of UHC in the UK.

We invited 11 highly experienced and respected healthcare academics, commentators, managers, clinicians, patient representatives and policymakers, to write contributions about how the future of UHC in this country might be safeguarded. All authors were given as their brief: 'Universal healthcare for tomorrow: If we were able to restructure British healthcare in any way we wished, how should it be changed?' The use of the phrase 'universal healthcare' in this brief was significant. We did not want authors to simply consider ways of saving the NHS in its present form. Rather, we wished them to formulate strategies to preserve all that the NHS stands for: namely, free and equal access to healthcare for the entire British population. As will be seen in the resulting chapters, many authors suggest that the battle for the continued viability of UHC in the UK rests beyond the existing healthcare services. Each invited contributor, by virtue of their expertise, was selected to bring an appropriate though differing approach to the issue, and was further selected as being representative of different political positions. Some were likely to be in favour of keeping the NHS as a single state institution while others might wish other parties to become involved in healthcare provision. Authors were informed that whatever they regarded as working well in the current system could be left unchanged or expanded, while any aspects they considered to be inefficient or harmful could be modified or removed. In short, we encouraged them to be as imaginative and creative as possible.

It is hoped that the resulting essays, from such varied yet well-qualified experts, might give policymakers with all levels of responsibility increased confidence in the implementation of seemingly radical ideas; ideas which could well prove vital to the successful future of UHC in this country. This introduction is not intended to be a collection of chapter highlights, instead it attempts to identify certain complimentary positions within the chapters and thereby sketch a cohesive narrative for the publication as a whole.

Public health and preventative medicine

No other themes are more frequently addressed in this book than those of public health in general (the health of the general population not using clinical services) and preventative medicine. A measure of their present comparative neglect is perhaps best summarised by David Hunter, who observes that 'the urgent forever drives out the important' in healthcare policy priorities, suggesting the NHS's struggle to maintain its present level of service leaves little time or financial resources to enable future planning. Phil Hammond likens the NHS's lack of preventative strategies to an attempt to rescue a never-ending stream of people from a river of illness. Science, he maintains, allows us to dive deeper and deeper; pulling out ever sicker individuals. However, this effort leaves the rescuers so busy that they have no time to move upstream and stop people falling into the river in the first place. Mark Porter and Sally Al-Zaidy take a similar view, arguing that society cannot continue to 'medicalise' all of its problems. Instead it must direct its efforts toward promoting good general health and preventing disease. John Ashton suggests that it might even be advisable to create a secretary of state for public health to counter the marginalisation and undervaluation of preventative initiatives.

Many authors highlight the importance of having a wider focus to healthcare than concentrating on health services alone. In addition, they suggest that society should have health-enhancing objectives in mind when considering policies in areas such as urban planning, education and employment. Such would be what Porter and Al-Zaidy term a 'health-in-all-policies' approach. Echoing this sentiment, Stephen Dorrell reminds us that 'public health is not a discrete service line; it is a way of thinking about public policy'. He believes Public Health England, established in 2013, must develop the institutional self-confidence to speak 'truth unto power' and call national governments to account for the health impact of its decisions across the range of its activities. 'No minister has the power to silence well-evidenced public health interventions,' he writes. Hunter holds that we might better understand public health in terms of either a community of interest with social and structural determinants of health, or alternatively as self-interested individuals seeking to make individual life changes.

Individual initiative and personal responsibility

This notion of individual choice of lifestyle, implying increased personal responsibility for health is a second important area of consensus amongst contributors. Corrigan likens the effort and perseverance of patients in improving and maintaining their health to that of hard-working students in improving their school's academic reputation: 'active patients', he holds, 'make better healthcare'. However, the idea of personal responsibility for one's health is, writes Richard Saltman, 'anathema to most defenders of the traditional English NHS', even though 'most providers know well that patients themselves take responsibility for and meet more than two-thirds of their medical needs'. Saltman believes that the wider British public, rather than just the medical and political community, must acknowledge that some diseases are not simply the result of bad luck, but are to a greater or lesser extent contracted due to an individual's own unhealthy behaviour.

Wherever the responsibility for disease might ultimately be held to lie, many authors suggest the future of healthcare looks likely to require an increased level of involvement from individuals in the maintenance of their own personal health. To allow this, healthcare itself may need to become more individualised and more integrated into daily life. While improvements to surgical techniques help the NHS make savings by ensuring fewer patients have to stay in hospital after procedures, and those that do for shorter times, Steve Melton holds that this is only a foretaste of what is to come; that 'technology emerging today makes science-fiction look backward'. Similarly, in his contribution, Marco Viceconti talks of the advance of existing predictive technologies linked to health. Such technologies will, he believes, provide personal health forecasting via portable sensors which can monitor the body's physiology and collect lifestyle data.

Such predictive technologies could flag up, with high certainty, future ailments likely to affect each individual if they do not modify their lifestyle, and even recommend effective health enhancing modifications to their behaviour. Viceconti believes this availability of immediate data and advice will help patients safeguard their personal health and enable them to make well-informed decisions when choosing between prospective treatments.

The introduction of personal healthcare budgets is also considered by some contributors. Corrigan believes such budgets could alter the balance of power in favour of the patient and away from politically and economically sensitive institutions like the NHS. However, he warns that the NHS might become 'dislocated' if patients were suddenly able to buy their own healthcare, potentially undermining the reason for the organisation's existence and that consequently the NHS is unlikely to adopt such an initiative of its own accord. However, as Melton predicts, 'future patients are more likely than any generation yet to be active consumers rather than passive recipients of care. They are used to making informed choices in most aspects of their lives.' It seems obvious that any such move towards the 'consumerisation' of healthcare would certainly pose a challenge to the fairly traditional structure of the NHS, but several chapters suggest the future sustainability of the organisation looks likely to be determined in part by the attitude taken towards it by its patients. Hammond reminds us that 'every day we don't have to use the NHS, someone who does, benefits. Those of us healthy at the moment have a responsibility to remain so for as long as we can'.

However, any consumer type attitude taken towards the NHS could not be the same as that taken towards the choice of homes, cars and holidays, as the utilisation or non-utilisation of the NHS unavoidably effects others. Whether a stable, universal healthcare system can be maintained in the long term without all members of society accepting more personal responsibility for their health seems far from certain. Any large-scale suggested change is likely to provoke debate concerning just how much socioeconomic inequalities and a lack of social cohesion are to blame for individual maladaptive behaviours; currently a matter of great contention across the political spectrum. As Corrigan writes, people undoubtedly do, to some extent, make their own health, 'but not under conditions of their own choosing'. He holds that society consequently has the responsibility to work with underprivileged groups to change these unfavourable conditions.

An enhanced role for civil society

Many authors advocate an enhanced role for civil society in healthcare. Melanie Reid, for example, expresses concern at so many different charity groups being involved in combating the same diseases such as cancer and heart disease. What needs to happen in the future, she suggests, is that charities should 'knock their heads together', share their knowledge, and end such strict specialisation in the allocation of their resources. She believes that by so doing they could play a far bigger role in providing care, especially for those suffering from chronic illnesses, with the state limiting itself to setting and policing minimum standards.

In a similar vein, Corrigan recognises the considerable benefit that might accrue from large patient organisations helping to provide services. Most such organisations 'have a deep knowledge of the day to day needs of their patients'. They also enjoy the trust of both patients and clinicians. In terms of primary care, Corrigan foresees a future healthcare system no longer solely directed by the NHS, but also with a major role played by patients, their families and local communities. Ashton, too, maintains that we need to move to an era where our health orientated associations are no longer 'co-opted' to fit the existing programmes of our institutions, but rather that the reverse occurs. The state's principle role in healthcare, he holds, ought to be one of mobilising and empowering communities to take action rather than simply patching people up when they become seriously or irreversibly ill. Indeed, as Saltman points out, much of the health and social care work in this country is given by informal caregivers, working independently of the NHS, anyway. He believes that state support for such caregivers should thus be made a priority, particularly in terms of readily available respite care and professionally staffed help-lines. Such an initiative would, he holds, enable many frail and elderly people to stay in their own homes longer, avoiding expensive residential care. 'Imagine if each of these people could live independently at home for an extra year' writes Ashton, citing the example of 10,000 dementia sufferers in Cumbria. 'That equates to 10,000 person years not spent in residential care home or hospital bed'. Such efforts have the potential to save considerable sums of health service money as well as giving many elderly patients an enhanced quality of life. Dorrell believes change lies in 'challenging the health and care sector (of which the NHS is an important part but not the whole) to deliver collaboration, not just with itself, but with the full range of local public services'. For example, he highlights how nonsensical it is to think about pediatric services without thinking about schools and children's social services also.

Mental health

Porter and Al-Zaidy emphasise the importance of establishing good healthcare in its fullest sense: that of complete physical, mental and social wellbeing. Hunter terms mental health as one of the 'wicked' public health problems that threaten the financial sustainability of the NHS. Ashton is of a similar opinion, identifying the prominent health problems of our age as being 'epidemic obesity and mental distress' with 'isolation, loneliness and depression in older age'. These he writes, are 'becoming ever more major public health issues' from which even younger people are not exempt in 'an increasingly fragmented and uncertain society'. Reid lists mental health amongst contemporary society's 'handful of unfortunate aces'; diseases, that she believes, might be treated by specialist independent hospitals supported by charities with only minimum state intervention. Such centres, she writes, could rapidly receive patients from A&E thereby relieving demand on the NHS's limited resources.

In order to better facilitate any proposals to improve mental health services, the need is recognised by some contributors to reduce the demand for them in the first place, as is equally the case with physical health ailments. Hammond, for example, talks of building up a mentally resilient population; a population with 'healthy minds as well as bodies'. As 'physical health stems from mental health', he writes, we need to create 'happy and resilient cities, communities and organisations that promote mental health if we want our individuals to flourish'. Richard Murray calls for a parity of esteem between mental health and other healthcare services, a proposal that has been widely discussed for many years without significant progress. Any strategy to improve mental health services, he holds, would need to be prepared for by a strategic shift in health workforce composition, the preparation for which would have to begin many years in advance.

Areas with a weaker consensus

Given the wide range of professions and various political persuasions among the authors, it is perhaps not surprising that there are a number of issues not agreed upon by the contributors. The independence of the NHS from political considerations is one such. Corrigan holds that the NHS owes its origin to a political manoeuvre and that consequently, we cannot expect it not to be inherently political. We cannot hope, he writes, to 'abstract' NHS policies from the 'messy business of politics'. Conversely, Murray believes that party political involvement has hindered the NHS from engaging in effective long-term planning and prevented the British public from understanding its goals and thereby effectively cooperating with it. Such political differences are apparent throughout the political and healthcare communities and could be why, despite various proposals over many years, no all-party group or committee dedicated to the NHS has ever materialised. Another reason might be that, even supposing such a group existed and could agree on policy, it would still be the government in power that would be held responsible for the success or failure of the committee's initiatives.

A second area lacking in consensus between authors is that of whether a purely publicly funded system can be expected to adequately meet the demands placed upon it now and in the future. Saltman believes that government policymakers really only have two economically viable choices for the future. The first is to continue the public financing of healthcare through taxation with the risk that, by an inability to raise already high taxes, the NHS might fall behind international standards of good healthcare. The second is to find the least socially damaging mechanism of collecting additional revenue from patients or citizens themselves. Melton takes a more conciliatory view of the same issue, holding that compared to other OECD countries, the UK government is 'neither absurdly generous, nor radically underfunding the system', and that it is 'almost pointless to say the NHS needs more money, because it is always going to need more if it is to meet future demand with the current system'.

On a third, contentious issue, of independent sector involvement, Reid believes that it is only nostalgia and sentimentality that are protecting the NHS from change, and that, like it or not, the NHS must adopt a mixed public/private funding strategy if it is to survive in anything like its current form. Opposing such a view, Porter and Al-Zaidy believe there exists no conclusive evidence that involvement from the commercial sector can offer improved services or even value for money. This debate is, however, not a new one. Dorrell finds it bizarre how the Blair government (in 2002) and the Coalition government (in 2012) both felt the need to re-legislate an idea that had 'been settled in government policy for over a quarter of a century'. Kenneth Clarke had proposed the introduction of a purchaser/provider split as early as the late 80s but, as Dorrell writes, this was ignored amidst 'the political noise' of these two subsequent proposals. While some contributors argue that competition and a profit motive are what British healthcare services need to raise their efficiency and effectiveness, others worry that a perverse incentive to profit might prove harmful. An example of this is the relative ease with which companies have been able to pull out of providing particular services when they become unprofitable, and the subsequent disruption to services caused. This publication cannot hope to offer any definitive conclusion to this long standing disagreement, there being seemingly cogent arguments on both sides, but at least it is hoped that by hearing the arguments the point at issue might become clearer.

Outside of the NHS

The overall structure of British healthcare can be likened to a rigid mould. Brand new, molten hot ideas are continually poured into it, ideas that seem beneficial and sometimes revolutionary. However, these ideas soon cool and assume the characteristics of our health system's existing structures. This is not to say that innovative ideas do not benefit the service, but as many contributors to this collection discuss, to improve such a colossal organisation as the British health service will take time if its stability is to be preserved. It needs to evolve rather than leap into its own future. The structure of British healthcare has long-established divisions with strict boundaries; boundaries that delineate acute hospitals from community care, primary care and public health services, and boundaries that isolate social care services altogether. Such specialisation and segmentation often generate excellence in particular areas, but it is frequently inflexible, restricting effective adaptation as the British population's needs evolve over time. 'The NHS risks being the classic sort of organisation that fails to champion change, even if it would benefit in the long term – simply because it is so focussed on what it does now,' writes Melton, citing by analogy Kodak's refusal to embrace digital photography and thereby hastening the company's failure in 2012. His point being that, in effect, it is often 'success that can prevent rapid change'.

Despite complete freedom on the part of contributors to alter or reject any aspect of our existing health service, each has resisted the temptation to lay out a brand-new healthcare utopia. The authors certainly suggest innovative, sometimes radical, ideas, proposing various means to reform this country's health services that they might function more efficiently in the future. However, most have focussed on an understanding of what good health and the responsibility for maintaining it might entail, both on a personal and institutional level, and have not suggested a complete overhaul of what presently exists.

When authors address specific healthcare services, they most often speak in terms of encouraging gradual, stable change. Hammond writes: 'I am loathe to suggest any structural miracle pill for universal healthcare. Continuous evidence-based improvement is far more likely to work, raising the quality bar a little at a time, as resources allow.' Melton echoes this view, arguing that local managers should be given 'licence to innovate', and that they be supported in taking 'sensible risks and trying new things'. This might prove more effective in improving the service, at least at the local level, than any large scale reorganisation. In every contribution a change of mentality on the part of politicians, medical staff, the public and patients is called for; that by altering the outlook of all interested parties, but where no one ideology dominates, effective and lasting improvement might be achieved. We need to 'look at changing culture', not just changing funding or structural issues, states Melton. From the collection of chapters in this publication it seems the issue for the 21st century will be not so much one of how the NHS should be redesigned, but one of what needs to be done at its fringes or even completely outside the organisation so that we might become less dependent upon it.

Typically, Murray writes: 'Whether by a possible tax on saturated fats, or regulations that can control access to alcohol, national policy making needs to show it has considered health in a more fundamental way'. Frequently, authors express confidence that predictive and preventative healthcare measures will become increasingly effective in reducing the need for acute medical interventions; a necessity because, as Viceconti states, 'healthcare is currently one of the only sectors where new technology increases instead of decreases costs'. In the past, the emphasis in healthcare development has generally been placed on offering interventionist treatments and cures linked to the marketing concerns of pharmaceutical research and allied industries. Fortunately, it now seems that researchers and companies are increasingly turning their attention to disease prediction and prevention. Rising public interest in personal health and wellbeing is leading this trend, as individuals become more aware of the risk that certain behaviours pose to health. Nevertheless, it is reassuring that, even if much healthcare innovation moves beyond NHS acute intervention services, the organisation is likely to survive in its present form. Medical emergencies will occur despite all efforts to promote good public health and human life is ultimately finite. As Murray states, 'the NHS has the support of the public of England, something few other countries can boast of having'.

Personally, I hope our publication will bolster the case for increased investment in improving these pre-clinical determinants of the health of the nation. If not, the NHS is likely to remain in crisis, faced with ever-increasing demand from a rapidly ageing population, often debilitated by extremely unhealthy lifestyles; a situation which threatens the service's stability and perhaps even its survival. Collectively, these chapters suggest that we need to wean ourselves from a total reliance on the NHS and become more mature in accepting a measure of responsibility for our own health and wellbeing.

A public health perspective

John Ashton

The arguments are, by now, well rehearsed. The British National Health Service is under attack as never before, squeezed on the one hand by a rapidly ageing population with increasing health needs, higher expectations and the much enhanced possibilities for evidence and science based interventions to make a difference; on the other by global economic forces, austerity and the longstanding ideological and political objections to publicly funded and provided services.

It is now more than two generations ago that the returning troops from the Second World War combined with the Home Front to create a cross-party consensus in favour of the creation of a welfare state. Having grown up during the long years of the recession of the 1920s and 1930s and seen off fascism, they were fired up by the need to create the conditions which would prevent a recurrence. The enemies now were want, ignorance, idleness, squalor and disease.[1] The weapons were social security, universal education, employment exchanges, town planning, a massive house-building programme and the National Health Service. The NHS itself was part of a public health service extending across local government and including family health and social services, dentists, opticians, pharmacies and general practice as well as hospitals. It is worth revisiting this context here because in the intervening years we have drifted imperceptibly from a health system grounded in public health to one in which healthcare, and in particular hospital care, has come to be seen as *the* system, with public health an increasingly marginalised and unvalued add-on.

As a public health practitioner my career has spanned almost exactly the period since the emasculation of public health in 1974, when the comprehensive approach which had served us so well for over 100 years was dismantled, until the present time when the return of public health leadership to local government and the setting up of a national public health agency still leaves us with a set of arrangements that are a shadow of their former selves, leaving the hospital, general practice and social care services to consume all of society's smoke. As I write, £200 million is proposed to be docked from the already tiny local authority public health budgets. So what is to be done?

We must, as ever, begin with the vision, without which the NHS will perish. Almost from its outset it has suffered from short-term meddling by each new set of politicians, anxious to make their mark. Structural change in the absence of functional understanding has been a monotonous feature of this meddling and we have paid a heavy price, not just in terms of costs but staff morale and most importantly the impact on population health. Unusually, the publication of the recent Five Year Forward View by the chief executive of the NHS, Simon Stevens, gives us a hint that the penny might have finally dropped – we can only hope so![2]

It is not as if there has been a lack of thought given to the vision around the world. For almost 40 years the World Health Organisation (WHO) has been advocating the need for health services to be reorientated to be based on population and public health principles. Beginning with the Alma Ata declaration in 1978,[3] leading to its 'Global Strategy for Health for All by the Year 2000' in 1981,[4] the WHO has been arguing the case for a fundamental shift of emphasis towards policies for prevention at a societal level with full public engagement, and systems built on primary healthcare with solid partnership working.[5] Some countries were actually listening. Finland, for example, took the decision 40 years ago to stipulate the proportion of health funding to be spent on prevention and primary care.[6] The mature Finnish system is worth a visit for anybody who wishes to touch and feel what the proper basis of a 21st century public health system can look like and the North Karelia Project for community control of heart disease remains an invaluable prototype over 30 years later.[7]

As for the wider determinants of health – those big issues so clearly defined by Beveridge and the other giants of the post-war period, such as Richard Titmuss who spoke of the importance of 'the control of resources through time' (not just money) – we have no excuse for a lack of awareness or understanding of what they are.[8] *The Black Report* in 1980 and a stream of reports and books on inequalities in health since,[9] culminating in Michael Marmot's recent publication *The Health Gap*, lay out the task in concrete detail.[10] The real question is whether any government has the political will to grasp the nettle when so many hostile forces are at play, not least commercial interests who by default hold sway over major areas of everyday life that impact on public health (processed foods, soft drinks, alcohol, tobacco, the motor industry, to name a few). It seems that too often we have lost sight of the lessons of history, one of the most important being that the health of the nation is not an optional extra but a prerequisite for national and economic success, whether in the Olympic stadium, on the cricket pitch or in the stock exchange, and sometimes on the battlefield. Who remembers today after more than 100 years of empire and huge tracts of the world being pink on the map, that around 30% of working class recruits were unfit for military service in the Boer War? The ensuing government enquiry in 1906 led to the establishment of the school health service, school meals and school milk. Military conflict with Germany loomed and we could take no chances. Today the parallels are clear. The world has become politically and economically more unstable than at any time since the 1930s and we are faced with epidemic obesity and mental distress.

To create that vision requires political will and real political leadership. The whole system change that is required needs to carry all sections of the community with it. The challenge in educational and communications terms is immense and trust is of the essence. Unfortunately, following on from the Lansley reforms and in the context of a government locked in dispute with the professions, it is in short supply. It is not helped by politicians manning the barricades in their own constituencies when essential reconfigurations are proposed. Above all we need a flourishing of health advocacy, debate and dialogue. The gagging of local directors of public health and the restricted scope of Public Health England to provide challenge are major impediments to the establishment of the open, participative culture of public health which is necessary. The vision must be one of a level playing field for health within a framework of corporate social responsibility. The propaganda about the 'nanny state' is not helpful here. The protection of the people's health and security is one of its primary responsibilities. We understand that with narcotic drugs and have come to understand it with regard to child and elder abuse, drunk driving, seat belts, food adulteration and many more issues. A blanket, knee-jerk phobia about government action to protect the individual against external threats must be tempered by an understanding of the benefits. Ironically the 'One Nation' Conservative party of the 19th century supported the development of a robust public health system at the local level within clear and progressive legislative frameworks. This is in marked contrast to the antipathy displayed towards legislative approaches at the present time which is not reflected internationally or nearer home in Wales.[11] One hopes that steps towards the implementation of the 'National Living Wage' represent the beginnings of the rediscovery of the government's central role in public health.

For public health leadership to be effective it needs a proper legislative framework and championing from the heart of government. There should be a secretary of state for public health within the Cabinet Office, a national director of public health who is fully and professionally trained in public health and the inter-departmental public health committee – introduced in 2010, but short-lived – should be brought back. Public Health England should be reinvented as a fully autonomous policy and advocacy body with a separate arms-length service arm and, at the local level, the Boards of Health and Wellbeing should be seen as what they really need to be – a 21st century reincarnation of local, integrated government, taking a strategic view of the public's health and wellbeing with pooled governance and funding, directly accountable to the public by election.

A prescription for action

The situation we find ourselves in is clear. In 1948, coming out of the war we faced a legacy of poverty, high unemployment and large families, many living in squalor and still with the residual threat of early death from childhood infections, tuberculosis and epidemic pneumonia. There was a deeply ingrained fear of the workhouse and the workhouse hospital, a fear of illness-induced debt and a lack of confidence in the 'panel' GP. The aspiration was of care in something akin to a voluntary hospital.

Much has changed 70 years on. The advent of the contraceptive pill transformed the options open to women as did the opening up of higher education opportunities, at least partially across the social spectrum. Fertility rates plummeted: from almost 1 million births in 1947 the annual cohort fell to nearer half a million before picking up again. However, in the round, the total period fertility rate is still below replacement level even when taking into account the slightly higher fertility of new Britons in recent years. Up to a fifth and more of women today have no children. At the other end of the spectrum, beginning in the 1970s, large numbers of people began to live into their 70s, 80s and beyond. This has been a result of improved living and working conditions, improved living standards coupled with the benefits of modern medicine, but it has not been equally distributed. Less advantaged families and communities still bear a disproportionate burden of avoidable ill health and preventable death.

These demographic changes have been accompanied by major social change which has implications for health, wellbeing and health and social care. For one thing, the traditional nuclear family is no longer the norm. Later marriage – if at all – and the prevalence of divorce have led to a surge in single-person and single-parent households. The movement of young people through higher education and the mobility of the labour market have led to a fragmentation of families and communities. Isolation, loneliness and depression in older age have become major public health issues together with the organic manifestations of neurophysiological decline, and younger people have not been exempt from the mental distress of an increasingly fragmented and uncertain society.

The institutional model of response, with the hospital at the centre and services focused on needs being met by ever more differentiated professional groups, is increasingly being seen as flawed. The future is going to be characterised by tensions which include that of specialist versus generalist, mono-discipline versus multi-discipline, and centralisation versus decentralisation. It will need to be horses for courses based on whatever evidence we can find.

Let's start at the whole population level. Commentators such as Ivan Illich,[12] John McKnight[13] and Lowell Levin[14] have long drawn our attention to the pitfalls of over-professionalisation and neglect of the intrinsic assets of individuals and communities.

Illich echoed George Bernard Shaw in seeing professions as conspiracies (against the laity), while McKnight pointed out that there was an abundance of skill and gifts in every community, that people are 'half full' rather than 'half empty', waiting for professionals to come along and 'fix them'. Levin has spoken of the 'lay health care system' of family, friends and neighbours which provides the majority of health and social care.[15] A person with Type 2 diabetes might spend a total of several hours each year in consultation with a medical adviser, the rest of the time they are 'It', needing to be their own health expert supported by their intimates and colleagues. But we have never sought to optimise this widely available resource which costs little and could be strengthened at modest cost. McKnight's group at Evanston University in Illinois has spent the past 40 years working in inner cities across North America and now globally and here in the north-west of England developing the approach known as asset-based community development (ABCD).[16] They have developed tools to be used by community organisers to enable them to map the individual, group, economic and environmental assets and connect them to institutional resources which can help them mobilise, grow and realise the potential of those assets.

McKnight draws the comparison between 'project funding', typically for three years, which requires a project bid for funds which must be spent by the end of the period, culminating in a further bid for funds for the next three years. The result is 'ugly contests' in which bidders must prove that they continue to be needy to merit outside intervention. Frequently such funds are used to pay for outside experts who come and go taking the money with them (as salaries) with the money never touching the sides of the communities through which it passes. In contrast, asset-mapping and mobilisation begins with the community's assets and by the end of the three years they have grown in many ways, not least in the legacy of empowerment. The challenge for institutions is to change the way they work so that they support the autonomy of individuals, communities and groups, rather than creating professional dependency. When I was working with the old Irish community based in the parish of 'Our Ladies' in north Liverpool (motto 'professionals should be on tap not on top') my public health education really began. They set about building their own housing cooperatives, employment opportunities, taking control of their environment and establishing a strong partnership for primary health care. When they began to secure large-scale funds for capital developments, they recognised the limitation of their financial expertise and I was able to secure the support of the finance department of the regional health authority to keep them on track.

In the village of Woolton in south Liverpool, an affluent suburb characterised by a high proportion of elderly people, the local senior partner in the health centre, Dr George Kuruvilla, became concerned about the numbers of elderly, especially widows, suffering from depression. He adopted an asset-based approach to the community and involved a wide range of community associations, including faith groups, in mapping the community assets. Building a substantial network of volunteers, they have published a directory of activities for use by the volunteers in engaging people in an active life in the community.

The social trends since the war have meant that whilst traditional communities still exist both within urban and rural communities, not least those which are ethnically or faith based, they are no longer universal. In my own experience in the context of Liverpool, the Vauxhall Catholics, the Yemeni and Arab communities, as well as the Jewish community, are exemplars of what can be done. However, even in country areas with the influx of suburbanites from the cities, facilitation for engagement may be needed even while there may still be a rich menu of country village life assets. The health centre or the school can be an important focus for building and supporting capacity for health and wellbeing through ABCD and community engagement. It may be the only meaningful point of organisational contact in a post-religious age.

The Coalition government in its early days proposed the 'Big Society'. In the event it appeared to be a case of the emperor's clothes. However, the work of McKnight and others has shown that it can have real substance. What it requires to make it happen is a network of community organisers based in schools, health centres, faith hubs and other relevant physical spaces. But it also needs the reorientation of professional working and the curricula and expectations of their professional bodies, of bureaucracies and institutions.

One major difference between traditional and contemporary communities may lie in the extent of the different types of social capital to be found within them.[17] In his seminal book, *Bowling Alone*, Robert Putnam distinguishes two forms of social capital, characterised by reciprocal action based on trust. Whereas bonding social capital is to be found within homogeneous social groups and is relatively easy to build, it is not always a good thing (think Klu Klux Klan).[18] On the other hand, bridging social capital is hard to build between heterogeneous social groups (think religion, ethnicity or social class), it is always a good thing. If we are real about strengthening the immunity foundations of resilience, solidarity and good health we must address these things. I see this as a challenge to the political left as well as the political right, in the same way that the strategic adoption of ABCD poses a challenge to unfettered capitalism as well as unfettered trade unionism.

Moving on from the whole population and a commitment to universal health development, I have already begun to make the distinction between 'associational' life (as McKnight calls it), and 'institutional' life which most professionals, public servants and employees inhabit. Associational life is characterised by flat, democratic arrangements, typically voluntary and focused around a matter of mutual concern and interest. In contrast institutional life is typically hierarchical and paid. Often, it is as if never the two shall meet, or if they do it is to see how associations can be co-opted to the mission of institutions rather than the other way around. We have seen this writ large in recent years as large voluntary organisations have been commissioned and contracted to provide big chunks of public sector work. This is usually very different from their origins as innovators and pioneers or as fillers of the cracks between statutory services. The challenge for the real 'Big Society' is to forge partnerships between associations and institutions based on mutual respect and understanding and where 1+1 can easily become three, four or five. The interfaces are really important but rarely addressed in a strategic and systematic way. Professionals are rarely familiar with the dynamics of working in an effective partnership with laity.

If we consider, for instance, the challenge of responding to dementia over the next 20 years, we will not do this without a plethora of scandals unless we can enable sufferers to live autonomous, participating and fulfilling lives within the heart of the communities they come from for as long as possible. This will require large-scale community mobilisation, coupled with the re-engineering and physical redesign of old housing and neighbourhoods and the establishment of norms for the new. I would quote the example of Cumbria, a county with which I am familiar having been the local director of public health for six years. Currently, there are over 6,000 people known to have dementia in a county of 500,000 people. Within 10 years it is expected that the number will be 10,000. Imagine if each of those people could live independently at home for an extra year! That equates to 10,000 person-years not spent in a residential care home or hospital bed. Think what that represents in financial and skilled human resources and then imagine how we could redesign everyday life and mobilise the community to make it unnecessary. It is possible but only with political will.

We are talking here of nothing less than transformation, and transformative thinking and leadership, which joins up our understanding of what it means in a salutogenic and health protective 21st century environment. It has implications for where and how we live, work, learn and play; for all professional groups and their professional bodies and training partners. If we are not to fall behind internationally we must start as a matter of urgency.

Turning to prevention, the community and lay care is critical to the future of the NHS, to primary care and the gateway into a budget of over £100 billion a year. The interface is of the utmost importance. Finnish colleagues have claimed that by systematically educating the public about their own management of common conditions, perhaps together with the local pharmacist, up to 20% of primary care consultations can be prevented. But have we ever tried to do this, in school or through the mass or social media? As for social media we are on a journey of unknown destination. The millennials (those coming of age since the year 2000) might as well be on a different planet from those of us who are older. Information and intelligence from social media drives their lives and professional opinion in person is increasingly a side show, yet it is still predominantly older people who are planning the future. It may end in tears unless we engage with the megastorms coming our way.

In this, primary care has itself been on a journey from the cottage industry of the traditional GP with his (sic) plate on the front door, taking patients as they turn up, via primary medical care with its teams of nurses and occasionally social work, increasingly aware of the practice list as a management tool, to primary health care in its full blown WHO public health orientated version. Probably the most highly developed model of this has been that of 'community-orientated primary care', as expounded by Kark and his group in Jerusalem.[19] With its origins in the Peckham Pioneer Health Centre in south London in the 1930s, via Johannesburg to Israel, this model is of place and population-based public health integrated into primary care, grounded in a local knowledge of epidemiology and health needs. It is a powerful model which has contemporary resonances around the world, not least in east London and parts of Cumbria. At its best it connects to the schools, faith communities, workplaces and much else. Tessa Jowell promoted it in part through the Healthy Living Centres of the Blair administration but they were short-lived and it is yet to see a mainstreaming by any government. As is often the case (e.g. Sure Start), sound initiatives fail to survive the vicissitudes of a change of government.

One of the strengths of community-oriented primary care is to make explicit the essential nature of strategic partnerships not only with other statutory agencies but with the voluntary sector. The advent of Boards of Health and Wellbeing over the past five years is one piece of structural architecture here which might be aligned with the necessary direction of functional travel, but only if this is also seen as part of the process of reform and strengthening of local government. The WHO Healthy Cities project, dating from 1986 and still going strong has sought to bring together many of the traditions of Victorian public health to the local level with its political mandate for concerted action on health.[20] Whilst Healthy Cities has created a global momentum for public health at the city, town and village level (person, place and governance), again it has never been mainstreamed. It is to be hoped that Andrew Stevens' endorsement of the Healthy Towns approach will finally enable Healthy Cities to enjoy central government support. If so it can provide a unifying framework for much of what we need to do and support the Five Year Forward View.

Public health (public mental health)

Around the world there is a growing recognition that we have been systematically neglecting mental health and the need for a public health approach to prevention, early intervention and continuing care. As measured by the burden of disease, mental ill health is now seen as a top priority and there is a growing campaign for parity of attention to mental and physical health.

The models for mental health and illness that we are working with are flawed and can never deliver what society needs to receive within the resources available. There will never be sufficient psychiatrically trained clinical staff to respond to the levels of distress or to get upstream to prevention. Even in the most generously funded public mental health services we are failing not only the needs of patients and their families but those of the wider society, the workplace and the economy. As Mao Tse Tung reputedly said: 'If the practice doesn't work the theory is wrong'.

Yet it doesn't have to be like this. Fifty years ago Gerald Caplan described an alternative approach – bottom-up and whole systems, grounded in public health.[21] A contemporary version of this would begin prenatally and follow the life course with full public and community engagement – not learnt through parents, teachers, schools and other community institutions – in which assets would be mapped and resources for resilience and good mental health mobilised. Strong clinical foundations would be found across the NHS but especially in primary care. A genuinely inclusive, multidisciplinary workforce would be developed across the clinical, educational and social sectors and specialist neuropsychiatric, biological and liaison input would have its scope clearly defined as a resource to a system that was built from the ground up. This is a huge challenge requiring vision and leadership and political commitment and support.

On intelligence

The basis of all public health is good intelligence and the availability of expertise to deploy it effectively. There is an urgent need for the building of epidemiological expertise and other methods of social and anthropological enquiry across public health and health and social care systems. Financial data and the current levels of management information available are insufficient as evidenced by recent scandals, including those at Mid-Staffordshire and Morecambe Bay hospitals. This expertise is needed across clinical and social services and beyond; it is needed at all levels. The need for it brings into focus the dysfunction inherent in training different public service leaders in separate tribal collegiate groups. The solution to this would be a network of public service staff training colleges which brought together future leaders from across the public services and equipped them not only with the transcendent technical and managerial skills for effective joint working, but also the transformational skills to achieve 21st century excellence.

The Five Year Forward View

The publication of the Five Year Forward View by NHS England in October 2014 provides a framework for action which is the best hope of reconciling the plethora of tensions surrounding public health and health and social care in an era of austerity. Seeking to avoid falling yet again into the trap of top-down structural reform whilst remaining strategic and not being lost in too many bottom-up flower beds blooming, seven new care models are proposed, all with the public and public health and prevention at their heart (see Table 1).

Table 1: New care models of the Five Year Forward View

1. Multi-speciality Community Providers (horizontal integration)

2. Integrated Primary and Acute Care Systems (vertical integration)

3. Urgent and Emergency Care Networks (appropriate centralisation-decentralisation)

4. Viable Smaller Hospitals (reconciling the needs of smaller communities with access to excellence in specialist care)

5. Specialised Care (centralisation-decentralisation/reconciling the needs of differing communities)

6. Modern Maternity Services (addressing the thorny issues of patient choice/geography, population density and patient safety)

7. Enhanced Health in Care Homes (addressing the issue of appropriate care closer to home and in the community, avoiding unnecessary hospital admission especially at end of life)

This menu provides a template for devolved services which is inherently a public health framework. The implications for all those involved in health leadership, whether as politicians, professionals and managers at local, regional or national levels are immense. There are many challenges for educational establishments and institutions. More of the same is not an option. Sir Derek Wanless's 'fully engaged' scenario is the starting point. So too is Charles Winslow's 1920 definition of public health as

> the science and art of disease prevention, prolonging life and promoting health and wellbeing through organised community effort for the sanitation of the environment, the control of

communicable infections, the organisation of medical and nursing services for the early diagnosis and prevention of disease, the education of the individual in personal health and the development of the social machinery to assure everyone a standard of living adequate for the maintenance and improvement of health.[22]

Postcards from the frontline

Melanie Reid

On a noticeboard in out-patients, in one of the many hospitals I frequent, is an action plan. One of the hospital's goals, it states, is:

'We aim for respect and dignity be 100% positive (sic)'.

And underneath, in the space for 'Actions', it says:

'As a result of your feedback we are working with the person centred collaborative in identifying and addressing real time areas of concern.'

To which the average patient, your tough, pungent Glaswegian, has one, absolutely correct, response.

'Whit the f*** does that mean?'

The WTF test is the cynical one-liner which cuts directly to the heart of the matter. I respect it hugely. I wish it could be applied across the board to this flawed monolith, the magnificent, dysfunctional, revered, anachronistic, socially-binding but bankrupt, life-saving institution we call the NHS. The NHS isn't just a health system, it is a world-famous cult. In 2010 I broke my neck (C6/7 incomplete) and became tetraplegic. I was an NHS inpatient for a year, latterly with weekends home for good behaviour. Subsequently I have been in hospital for three more operations, in various emergency, high dependency and acute wards, meaning another month or so inside. I have, you might say, lain and observed the essence of the NHS and its daily workings for somewhat longer than your average NHS accountant, manager or politician. (I had procedures in private hospitals too, so I am familiar with the alternative.)

My experience ranged from amazing to pretty abysmal. The service saved my life and restored me to a new existence, at God knows what cost. Undoubtedly a six figure sum. Enough to make an insurer cough, were it not for the fact that private medicine as presently constituted cannot treat traumatic spinal injury. Now, as someone who will suffer chronic disability for the rest of my life, I observe everything from primary care to hospital outpatient processes. I write this from a perspective of fond respect for the NHS, that great 'person centred collaborative' of the noticeboard, but also with the conviction that change is unavoidable.

There has to be a new funding mechanism

It's 7.30am and 15 of us have arrived at the colorectal ward for our on-the-day elective surgery. We're a mixed bunch: bowel cancer, Crohn's, hernias, colostomies. Most of us rose at 5am to get here and we're nauseous from fasting, on top of our usual misery. I've been waiting six months for this. The colorectal surgeon is one of the busiest men I have ever met.

By noon, wilting, whey-faced, some have been taken for surgery, others sent home. I have been quizzed by three consecutive nurses with forms, asking dozens of repetitive, unfathomably unnecessary questions. Has a GP ever warned me I am at risk from CJD infection?

An hour later, I too am sent home. There is no bed. 'I'm sorry; it's quart into pint pot every single day,' says a medic. I am one of around 80,000 people annually whose long-planned operations are cancelled like this, in almost every case from lack of resources. During the quarter ending 30 June 2015, in England and Wales, 16,180 operations were cancelled at the last minute for non-clinical reasons by NHS providers.[1] In Scotland no official figures are kept, but 30 cancellations a day are estimated.

The shortfall is built into the system. Every day hundreds of chronically ill people are led up the hill then all the way back down again. There are no statistics for the resultant human misery.

Simple, isn't it? I would like a health service which delivers what I need and does not make me suffer more than I already do. I would happily take out insurance for major expenditure and pay £10 every time I need to consult a GP. I want poor people to be reimbursed fully and everyone else on a sliding scale. I want tax for healthcare to be hypothecated. The basis for everything I suggest below predicates on the assumption that the NHS must invent some kind of private/public model. Like it or not, the public will have to start contributing. The system is no longer sustainable and simply increasing its budget every year, pretending this is the answer, is deceitful. There are not enough beds, surgeons, nurses, ambulances. Besides, however big the increase, it is now evident the money will never meet the massive demands posed by a) people living longer, with more chronic conditions; b) the speed (and expense) of technological advances in medicine; c) the expectation of patients that the latest advances and drugs will be available to them; and d) the threat of unforeseen events, such as failure of all antibiotics. Politicians of every party know this; everyone in the UK with half a brain knows it. There is, however, a nostalgia, a sentimentality, which keeps the NHS protected. One day, however, a government is going to have to risk annihilation at the polls by being the first to finesse the powerful myth of 'free' healthcare, and we can be sure of one thing: that whichever administration then succeeded, it would not reverse those reforms. For sure, the incomers would pretend to: tinkering at the edges, and rebadging, but that first step towards a contributory system, once initiated, would not be repealed. Because it is the only way.

In the knowledge, then, that turkeys will never vote for Christmas, I would suggest that some independent device is given the remit to explore this. I am not sure if royal commissions carry the immense gravitas they once did; I fear Chilcot has rather done for inquiries. Perhaps some prestigious new vehicle, some Bugatti Veyron of impartial wisdom and judgement, could be devised for this purpose, with cross-party support. Whatever happens, there is an absolute necessity to extricate the NHS from party politics and achieve some kind of consensus. To leave unexamined a failing but vital national institution, and allow it to be 'weaponised' every five years, is a betrayal of public duty, and therefore the nation.

I am no expert in the funding of other countries' health services. I am aware only that other European countries of similar wealth do it better and more cheaply than us, and the standard of care is generally lower for people of all incomes in the United Kingdom by comparison.[2] This is surely one reason alone why we need to change. France spends more on health as a percentage of GDP than the UK but has lower public expenditure (77% of total; UK 83.2%); more doctors (3.3 per 1000 population; UK 2.8); more MRI scanners (7.5 per million population; UK 5.9); a shorter wait for elective surgery (7% wait more than four months; UK 21%); better life expectancy (81.5; UK 80.6); and lower infant mortality (3.5 per 1000 live births, UK 4.2 per live births).[3] Anecdotally, from the French side of my family, and from passing personal experience, I would suggest that the French system, using a national programme of social health insurance, has indeed achieved that 'pragmatic blend of consumer choice, professional autonomy, central regulation and a government-backed guarantee for the poor, which exceeds the NHS standard on many counts.[4]

Fundamental funding reform of the NHS will be a massive PR task, above all else. In this the French system is a good model, if only because those Beveridgean ideals suit the liberal conscience. Its compulsory social health insurance (NHI) is managed almost entirely by the state and publicly financed through employee and employer payroll contributions and earmarked taxes. For the majority of patients, medical goods and services are not free at the point of use – patients pay an up-front cost which is partially and usually immediately reimbursed by the government. Critically, however, universal access is guaranteed by schemes for those on low incomes and/or chronic conditions. For areas not covered by NHI, there is a voluntary private health insurance (VHI) sector.

Some examples of NHI reimbursement rates: typically 80% of the cost of hospital treatment, although there is a daily charge of €18 for stays over 24 hours; 50-75% of GP visits; 65-100% of vaccinations; 35-100% of prescriptions; 30% of transport costs. There are some recent co-payments which are not reimbursable by either NHI or VHI and are intended to improve patient cost-consciousness without causing great financial strain. These co-payments are limited to an annual ceiling of €50 and include: €1 per doctor visit, €0.50 per prescription drug and €18 for hospital treatment above €120.[5] Similar contributions in Britain would improve the NHS; they would also be a fundamental step towards encouraging the public to accept more responsibility for their health. Significantly, the acceptance of a contributory model in Germany, like France, means that citizens and their employers take some responsibility for their healthcare, rather than leaving power almost exclusively in the hands of the state. And in France, there is anecdotal evidence that co-payment acts as a brake on consumption.

The care of chronic illnesses must be revolutionised

The reception at X-ray and ultrasound is packed with the long-term chronically sick. A grey-faced woman, probably only in her late 50s, is sitting wheezing for breath. A younger man, his dog tied on a string outside, is talking to himself, suffering either from alcohol or psychosis or both. Another woman, her skin vivid yellow against her dyed black hair, stares into the middle distance. There is an elderly couple, both with walking aids, their frailty terrifying. Resignation is set on our faces. People like us spend our lives waiting, retelling our stories to different members of staff.

A nurse arrives to summon someone; she is morbidly obese. Her 5XL uniform strains over her body; beads of sweat from the effort of moving cling to her top lip. She is young and has a beautiful face but her hips struggle to roll one vast thigh in front of the other.

I'm paralysed, but right now I'm feeling healthier than anyone.

Key to my NHS is the devolution of chronic illness into specialist hospitals, enterprises to be run jointly by charities and the private sector, with minimum standards of care set and policed by the state. These specialist centres would, as much as possible, be satellites around the emergency and acute hubs on the sites of big hospitals. The big six chronics are cancer, heart disease, strokes, diabetes, dementia and obesity, but add to that arthritis, COPD, hypertension, mental ill health, epilepsy, asthma and substance abuse, and you pretty much hold the handful of unfortunate aces. The chronically sick are the future. About 15 million people in England have a long-term condition like this, managed by drugs and other treatment, and their number is expected to double over the next 20 years. By 2018 the number of people with three or more long-term conditions is predicted to rise from 1.9 million to 2.9 million. People with long-term conditions now account for about 50% of GP appointments, 64% of outpatient appointments and over 70% of all inpatient bed days. The treatment and care of us chronics is estimated to take up around £7 in every £10 of total health and social care expenditure.[6]

Let's take the example of diabetes. The number of people living with the condition has soared by nearly 60% in the past decade.[7] More than 3.3 million people have some form of the disease, up from 2.1 million in 2005. Roughly 90% of cases are type 2 diabetes, the form closely linked to diet and obesity, which causes an inability to control the level of sugar in the blood, can lead to blindness and amputations and is a massive drain on NHS resources.[8] Diabetes, then, is inextricably linked to obesity. Sugar poses as much of a threat to national health as cigarettes.[9] In the UK, 67% of men and 57% of women are either overweight or obese. If obesity rates were to continue unchecked, it is estimated that 60% of adult men, 50% of adult women, and 25% of children in the UK could be obese by 2050[10], with a potential cost of around £50 billion. It is predicted that the annual NHS cost of the direct treatment of diabetes in the UK will increase to £16.9 billion over the next 25 years, which is 17 per cent of the NHS budget,[11] believed to potentially bankrupt the NHS.[12]

Charles Jencks, with his former wife, founded Maggie's Centres to act as charitably-run cancer support units. He has put forward a similar theory, suggesting every hospital needs separate, semi-autonomous, privately-run centres to care for patients with chronic diseases.[13] Not only would this relieve hospitals of a crippling financial burden, it would allow acute care to get on with the job it has to do. Critically, it would raise the quality of life for chronic sufferers exponentially, treating their complex mix of physical, emotional, social and financial issues.

My belief is that specialist centres should take responsibility for chronic patients at all stages. Emergencies could be triaged at A&E, then swiftly passed across for specialist care. Both the centres and the A&E hub would have acute wards but patients would move out of the hub for specialist post-op rehabilitation, physiotherapy and emotional and lifestyle support. Charity and insurance-funded, the specialisms would also deal with all non-emergency referrals, scans, diagnosis and follow-up.

Bariatric surgery, for instance. The patient would go to the bariatric centre, be appraised, and initially put on a supported (that word's crucial) lifestyle rehabilitation programme. Should that fail, the patient would then be referred to the hub for stomach stapling, joint replacement etc. After the operation, they would return to the bariatric centre for multi-disciplinary support.

I have experience of such a system already operating within the NHS. I spent a year in the Queen Elizabeth National Spinal Injuries Unit, in Glasgow, which under the vision of the recently retired orthopaedic surgeon David Allan was developed into a bold, multi-disciplinary specialist unit – anecdotally regarded as one of the best of its kind in the UK. QENSIU has under one roof a high dependency ward, effectively intensive care, for spinal patients; a rehabilitation ward; a gym with specialist physiotherapists; a therapy pool; a bioengineering and research unit; occupational therapist specialists in tetraplegic hands; specialist charity-run IT support; on-hand social workers; even a dedicated psychologist. There are fertility clinics and home visits, and liaison with local councils. Patients remain on the unit's books for life and have allocated liaison nurses. If more specialist care is needed – urological, colorectal, orthopaedic, neurological, gynaecological – then the unit will refer to consultants in the main hub hospital who have experience of spinal patients. They are even getting their own specialist Horatio's Garden.

This set up works impressively, perhaps because the unit manages to some extent to be self-governing and quietly dodges some of the worst of central NHS bureaucracy. When things were bumpy at QENSIU, in my observation as a patient, it was because the dead hand of the non-specialist NHS had interfered.

Of course the unit lacked staff and outpatient physiotherapy, but I will return to that later.

Imagine how consumer-friendly, economical and high-achieving a similar, multi-disciplinary centre could be for, say, bariatrics, diabetics and heart disease. In France, specialism flourishes at a decentralised level. A woman in a small town goes to a private local clinic to see her gynaecologist when she wants. In Germany specialism is built into the system. Disease Management Programmes are a form of insurance-organized, managed care instrument designed to improve coordination of care for chronically ill patients.[14]

It is worth stressing how care of patients is transformed by centres of excellence. Treatment is educated, resourced, tailor-made and sympathetic. Patients whose lives are miserable, who feel they are a permanent nuisance, may for the first time get a sense of being among people who *understand*. It is surely not too much to aspire to.

This is particularly true of mental health specialist units which would no longer be a Cinderella service. Future quality of life after strokes, for example, would also be improved by having stroke units attached to A&E to ensure that within four hours – the golden time period – victims can receive expert attention.

Emergency care must be freed up

The distressed elderly lady was admitted to my medical ward via A&E in the middle of the night. As the primary carer of her husband, who was dying of terminal cancer, she was distraught that she had had to leave him. Her body had betrayed her: she had collapsed in a flood of faeces and vomit and her daughter had called an ambulance.

She had been cleaned up and a stressed junior doctor was trying to take a blood sample. He could not find a vein, puncturing both her arms for the best part of 45 minutes. I lay in the dark listening to the harrowing soundtrack. It shouldn't be like this, I thought.

Few people would disagree that one of the things the NHS does best is saving imperilled lives. I propose that A&E should keep doing this, and remain entirely publicly funded, to ensure that expertise and speed of response in every unit conforms to nationally high standards. A&E staff would be better paid and the ethos would be, treat first, seek insurance policy numbers later.

But A&E at the moment is overwhelmed by people who shouldn't be there – those who cannot find a GP; the elderly, like the woman above; and people who have abused alcohol or drugs. The minute such people are discovered not to be at risk of death, the struggle is to find them a bed elsewhere, and clear space in A&E.

My intention is that A&E would be released to function at its life-saving best, if patients like my unfortunate lady above could be first triaged and then steered immediately to a specialist geriatric unit (as I expand on below). Similarly the drunks and addicts who fill A&E at night-time in big cities. They require specialist help, not life-saving intervention. Emergency medicine would flourish if such patients could be diverted fast to relevant units – and, from the patients' perspective, how much more expert would be their care.

Old age has to become a multi-disciplinary speciality

I am lying, this time, in an acute orthopaedic ward in one of the biggest teaching hospitals in Europe, recovering from an emergency operation to repair a broken hip and, a few days later, an elective colostomy.

It's fair to say I am not a typical patient. The rest of the beds are filled with old ladies, bird-like creatures who have fallen and broken their hips: their prognosis is harrowing. Up to 10% will die within a month and up to 35% within a year.[15] A high percentage of them already had dementia and have come from care homes. In considerable pain, they scream and curse the nurses. I overhear staff trying to explain to them that there are no beds available at the geriatric unit or their local care home, so they must stay here. The few who are not demented quickly succumb to urinary infections and become hallucinatory. My neighbour, bright as a button when admitted, slowly fades into deep confusion, apathy and weakness as the days pass post-op. Physiotherapists give her the mandatory brutal sessions: up on her feet on her new hip the next day. But she's too weak. They have to leave her in bed from where she may never rise.

When a bed does become empty, it is filled within two hours. A mountaineer is brought in, flown to A&E by helicopter. She has broken a leg badly. But the next day, operated on and heavily plastered, she goes home. Only the pitiful elderly remain – the demonised 'bed-blockers'.

I'm still here because I'm waiting for a bed at the spinal unit, for physiotherapy to allow me to continue normal wheelchair life. Plainly nobody has told the registrar. He approaches my bed - like many an orthopod, he's best dealing with people under anaesthetic.

'Why are you still here?' he says crossly. 'Do you know this acute bed is costing £400 every day? We need it.'

We know well that the present infrastructure cannot cope with the future burden of an ageing society. It has been demonstrated that:

- Using hospital beds more efficiently could save the NHS at least £1 billion a year and deliver benefits for patients.

- More than 70% of hospital bed days are occupied by emergency admissions.

- 10% of patients admitted as emergencies stay for more than two weeks, but these patients account for 55% of bed days.

- 80% of emergency admissions who stay for more than two weeks are patients aged over 65.

- Reducing the length of stay for older people has the most potential for reducing hospital bed use.[16]

Hip fractures alone cost the UK an estimated £5 million per day – that is £2 billion per year.[17] The cost to treat one hip fracture is £13,000 in the first year and £7,000 for the subsequent year.[18] So it is a sad situation. Hospital beds will continue to be occupied by the frail and elderly longer than they should be; and the absence of suitable beds elsewhere will eventually overwhelm the NHS. My proposed specialist geriatric units, therefore, would be run with public/private/charitable money, but also local authority budgets, thus uniting social and health care for the elderly. Keeping the two systems apart and separately funded no longer makes sense (if it ever did).

My geriatric centre of excellence, then, will receive elderly people from everywhere – A&E and elsewhere. It will assess, rehabilitate and arrange suitable longer-term residential care if the patients are unable to return home. There could also be specialist hospice units, offering the best and most dignified end of life care. Given that old age is an enormous, complex area of medicine, nursing and social demand, these centres would offer a multi-disciplinary care which would I hope go some way towards redressing health inequalities for the elderly. There would be focus on the individual – on rehabilitation, occupational therapy, and a prioritising of the need for independence. Is it too much to hope the units would be cheerful, sunny places which would reverse some of the decades of prejudice and neglect of the frail elderly?

The warm fuzzy feeling must be preserved

Working in a spinal unit isn't for everyone: a big percentage of every day requires clearing up adult faeces. Paralysed bowels are fun neither to possess nor care for.

One of the warmest, cheeriest nursing auxiliaries is a single mother from the toughest of areas, striving to get her children into college. She works 12-hour shifts on the minimum wage to hold her household together, 12 intense hours of hard, smelly labour, run off her feet. She brings light and humour to the angriest patients, who grumble and swear and ring their buzzers incessantly.

If the unit is ever short-staffed, they phone her up and she drops what she is doing and comes on shift. On one of her days off, she travelled into the city centre to buy a special T-shirt for a young man newly paralysed.

'I love this place,' she says. 'I feel part of something special.'

That warm, fuzzy feeling is the NHS's greatest asset. Best described as a mixture of pride, altruism, generosity and compassion, it is the impulse that the best NHS staff have to help anyone in distress, regardless of their circumstances. *It's what we do. It's what we're good at. We might have very little, personally, but we are professionals offering you everything. Our jobs, working for the NHS, give us importance and status.*

We welcome anyone. We belong to something great. As a result, kings and commoners alike get treated, mostly, with courtesy and kindness. As a form of unwritten morality, this attitude demands huge respect.

The public's attitude is similar. Their warm, fuzzy feeling is in the sense of ownership of the NHS. *It's free because it's ours.* For many people, this also brings a rather dangerous sense of entitlement – entitlement to the best of treatment, to decent meals, to shorter waiting times. Which also means an entitlement to moan when these things are not delivered.

How then to retain that warm, fuzzy feeling amongst the staff, that sense of open-armed generosity to allcomers; and also persuade the public that they will have to contribute personally to something they think they have already paid for? How not to damage what is, in its best form, a lovely relationship between staff and patients?

The basic humanitarian ethos of unquestioning free care, of embracing whatever sickness or disaster or disease is cast by the tide upon the doorstep, is profoundly admirable. It is what, as Sir John Tusa said of the BBC,[19] makes the NHS principled, idealistic, responsible and decent. To which we might add, and totemic to voters. If Britain tops a so-called global league for 'soft power',[20] then it is partly down to the reputation of the NHS.

The NHS staff are its greatest asset, but one under threat with overwork. Not only do they need nurturing, and better pay where the market demands it – rural GP practices; some unpopular consultant posts – but there needs to be a vital exercise in recognition. Were those things done intelligently, and people made to feel more valued and better treated, then the warm, fuzzy feeling can be preserved and absence records improved. (I'm not being over-idealistic here – the mediocre and lazy staff, who escape censure now, need recognition of a different sort.)

Staff must be re-empowered

The NHS reminds me of a communist state in miniature. Here's an example: Friday night and the heating has packed in. The ward is freezing; the ducts are emitting a screeching noise. At about 11pm, three hours after they were alerted, NHS in-house maintenance men arrive. Leisurely. There are five of them: wearing boiler suits and superior expressions. Their MO ranges from slow to stop. They ignore the patients completely. After a long pause while they get a ladder, one man climbs into the roof space through a ceiling panel; the other four stand at the foot of the ladder, jobsworths in a comedy sketch. 'Nah, Wullie,' says the man up above. 'It'll need to wait until Monday.' And so it does.

It strikes me the centrist tendencies of the NHS, over decades, have disempowered and de-incentivised staff. Much of this springs from the defensive culture of watching one's back against the threat of litigation. Some of the greatest managerial stupidities I have ever seen were in hospital, the result of an impossibly over-regulated bureaucracy which oppressed staff to the point where initiative is seen as a dangerous characteristic. Play it safe; tick the boxes; abide by the protocols; make no decisions. The result is monstrous amounts of unnecessary paperwork for all but the lowliest staff, and a general atmosphere of stasis. Simultaneously, management seeks to practise economies at the same time as it enforces an almost criminal level of institutionalised waste. Powerful organisations within the organisation – infection control, health and safety, protocol-setters, learning and development enforcers – operate almost like secret police units, setting ridiculous standards and causing life at the sharp end almost to seize up. They wield so much power that certainly in my experience no one could question their empire building. In reality, daily life functioned despite them. The good staff basically ducked and dived and bent the rules to get things done; the lazy staff would call in the union rep if they spied anyone using their initiative.

To thrive, hospitals must free their workforce from self-propagating bureaucracy. Nurse training needs to be revolutionised to liberate students from protocol and allow initiative to flourish. Working life in the NHS has an Alice in Wonderland logic, whereby, for instance, physiotherapists had to stop treating patients early in order to fill in timesheets justifying every 15-minute chunk of their working day... spent treating patients. Nurses could not leave the nurses' station and attend to patients because of the volume of unnecessary paperwork and emails pinning down every movement, every decision. Is it any wonder nursing students, brainwashed by rules and unaware what decision-making means, are less impressive than older nurses?

I witnessed many wasteful insanities enforced by infection control inspectors. Patients were dispensed drugs in sturdy plastic beakers, eminently washable, but which must be thrown out. Heavy plastic sliding sheets – to satisfy the moving and handling inspectors – must be thrown out after single use. Physiotherapists' electric plinths, when they were retired from NHS service, must be scrapped instead of being recycled to developing countries – because corners of the plastic upholstery were sometimes worn, which might lead to infection being passed on, and resulting litigation. Ditto old beds and ditto perfectly good expensive wheelchairs which, when replaced, were not recycled to countries in need because they could not be guaranteed safe for reuse.

Fear of litigation, from patients but also from their own staff, clogs the arteries of the NHS. And fear of litigation, like fear of censorship, is far more toxic than the concept itself. Health and safety regulations lead to staff being infantilised and patient care being hindered and compromised. There were almost laughable restrictions, under moving and handling rules, which taken to their ultimate would debar a nurse acting alone from helping a patient sit up, let alone help them off the floor should they slip. In 2012, after a civil action was lodged against NHS Highland at the Court of Session in Edinburgh, a nursing auxiliary received £50,000. She said she had suffered an injury to her neck and shoulders when curtains around a hospital bed jammed, and was unable to return to work after the incident.[21]

These are not just newspaper stories. There must be a better way of doing things; and surely, surely, we can ban adverts for personal litigation solicitors from hospitals.

I would like to preserve one of the best bits of communism – the idea that a big organisation contains a job for everyone, however lowly, with proper training. Some of the porters in the NHS are tough, scarred, tattooed, inarticulate men who would scare you if you met them on a dark night. Some are so rough they may never progress further. But I personally love it when I approach a reception desk and behind it is a tough-guy with full-sleeve tattoos, who confounds all expectations and turns out to be the most helpful person you meet all day. The NHS, however funded, must continue to offer people a route up.

It is also essential that staff are provided with gyms, crèches and major incentives to exercise, get well and lose weight.

Salami slicing no more

In the spinal unit, in order to save a few pennies, staff were supplied from central stores with a new, cheaper make of overnight urine collection bags (which are single use). Every night, at least two or three bags would burst, flooding the wards with urine. Hard-pressed nurses and auxiliaries had to spread incontinence pads (an oncost) on the floor; their other work was delayed; cleaners had to be called in. What it did to staff morale was probably most damaging of all.

Then there were the blankets. Or rather, there weren't the blankets. Central laundry was frequently unable to cope with supply and demand: some nights patients lay and shivered. In one major hospital my cousin, in a freezing single room, was told there were no blankets available. She placed her working farm jacket across her shoulders and asked her daughter to bring in a duvet. The nurses told her to remove them, declaring them an infection risk. Only by appealing to the consultant did sense prevail.

Salami slicing leads to false economies. Take the farce over the new-style, cheaper nurses' uniforms, universally procured, which were introduced in NHS hospitals in 2010/11. Instead of having buttons or zips down the front, these were over-the-head, extremely unflattering V-necks. Well might horrified staff point out that in the case of contamination, the garments would have to be pulled over their faces in order to change. It mattered not. Nurses with heavily soiled uniforms must now cut them off and throw them out, incurring greater cost in the future.

Make physiotherapy a priority

*After I left the spinal unit, where I received four hours of in-patient physiotherapy **a day**, I went to one hour **a week** from a community physio: this was traumatic. My achingly slow rehabilitation – the same goes for sufferers of strokes, brain damage and other neurological conditions - didn't just stall, it regressed. My body seized up. Specialist private neurophysiotherapy cost me £60 an hour, plus travelling time, for a home visit. Who can afford as often as they need it? In despair, my husband and I bought a Norwegian-made machine called a Topro Taurus, which, it is no exaggeration to say, has been life-changing. I have used it every day since and it has saved both my sanity and my body. It stands me up and enables me, with the help of one person, to practise walking. The Topro Taurus, battery operated, under £2,000 to buy, is a brilliant machine, but no NHS therapist I have ever spoken to has seen or used one. Every therapist who has seen mine has raved about it. How many other superb devices like it are languishing, unexploited, because they cost too much to contemplate? In a properly funded world, every geriatric and stroke centre would have multiple Topros, or similar.*

If there is one glaring need in the NHS, it is the shortage of sufficient out-patient physiotherapy. Patently, physio is regarded as a non-essential service and is cut to the bone. After all, people don't die if they get stiff and weak. But physical rehabilitation, for millions, is the key to recovery, quality of life and lower reliance on other NHS services. It is fundamental to a healthier population.

Patients with strokes, heart disease, diabetes, obesity, broken bones and neurological conditions, to name but a few issues, leave hospital after receiving brief in-patient physio. They go home and fall down the gap, because the provision of physiotherapy in the community is poorly resourced (for the same reasons: it's not life-saving). The process of recovering faculties, strength and movement, which goes on for years, is halted overnight.

Exercise and physiotherapy are key priorities for preventative work in public health. They reduce demand for services. My NHS would site specialist out-patient physiotherapy services in every single chronic illness centre. I would also fund community physiotherapy centres, perhaps based in local gyms, where stroke victims and disabled people, or MS patients eager to remain mobile as long as possible, can go every day if they are motivated enough. Out-patient hospital physiotherapy appointments should continue indefinitely for the chronically ill – a kind of lifelong drive to maximise better health. The physiotherapy would be funded as part of the whole private/public package; insurance companies could even incentivise people by offering them discounts if they attended physiotherapy-based courses.

Exercise should also be a fundamental part of mental health treatment.

Tackle the unsexy: urinary infection and incontinence

The ultimate Cinderella of the NHS is urinary infection and incontinence. The world of technology has bypassed this problem scandalously. The indwelling urinary catheter, unchanged in basic design for 80 years, is the most common cause of infections in hospitals and other healthcare facilities.[22] Urinary tract infections (UTIs) are tied with pneumonia as the second most common type of healthcare-associated infection. Virtually all healthcare-associated UTIs are caused by instrumentation of the urinary tract.[23] The cost implications of the neglect of this issue are mind-boggling. Anecdotally, community district nurses estimate 30% of their time is spent on catheter or urinary problems. The prevalence of urinary incontinence rises with age and creates major medical, social and economic problems. In 1998 the cost of incontinence to the NHS in England alone was estimated to be about £354 million; staff costs amounted to £189 million with aids such as pads and appliances such as catheters contributing £27 million and £59 million respectively. Using those figures, the total adjusted cost to the NHS in the UK would have amounted to c.£550 million in 2011.[24] The problem is hidden from view and dealt with on a short-term basis. In a publicly funded health system, such as the United Kingdom, there may be disagreements on where to invest, particularly when the opportunity cost of investing in one health innovation means that less money will be spent on some other health innovation.[25] Tackling urinary issues and modern solutions to catheters are a fundamental step to rebuilding the NHS.

Knock charities' heads together

At a conservative estimate, most big health issues have four or five charities all dedicated to helping sufferers. My own area has Spinal Research, Aspire, Back Up, Wings For Life, Spinal Injuries Association, Spinal Injuries Scotland. Each with a mission, a CEO, deputies, infrastructure and literature. Not to mention the host of smaller spinal charities, operating more locally or in the name of individuals. The number of cancer charities must run into three figures. This, in my opinion, is madness. The charities should be incentivised to unite, share resources, costs and infrastructure. Yes, by all means meet slightly different needs, but do so under an efficient, cohesive umbrella which would allow professional funding arrangements with the state and the private sector, in order to run the best, most tailored specialist treatments.

Future proof health services

In 2010 NHS Scotland opened the £300m state-of-the-art Larbert hospital. I was referred there in 2012 for a bone scan after I broke my hip, post paralysis. I was ushered into a small room containing the machine, and then told that they were very sorry, but they were unable to scan people in wheelchairs. The machine did not lower far enough for me to transfer onto it from my chair; there was not enough space to deploy a hoist to lift me.

My GP wrote to the hospital, despairing that people in wheelchairs were most at risk from bone thinning. They wrote back, apologising, but offering no alternative.

These are obvious things:
- Disability awareness has to be built into the core of the NHS. It is one of the certainties we can plan for, with an ageing population and one increasingly diabetic and obese.

- People must be made aware of their responsibility to their own health. Educating them in diet and exercise should be hard-wired into all government policy.

- Tackling the food and drink industry. Sugar is endemic in processed food. Fizzy drinks ditto. There are other dangers – a professor of incontinence told me that people in their twenties, addicted to the caffeine in fizzy drinks, are suffering increasingly from irritable bladder syndrome – the sudden urge to urinate. They face a stark future of incontinence from an early age.

And there are the less obvious:

- We can guesstimate how progressive developments may transform the future of healthcare – surgical robots, 3D printers and diagnostic machines are just the ones we have heard about. There will be more, with unquantifiable cost implications.

- Equally, we cannot predict what could happen in terms of *regressive* developments – for example the next zoonotic disease to replace ebola, with the possibility of a more terrifying result. Unexcitable veterinary academics have quietly been predicting a future Armageddon for some years now. And then there is the pressing issue of finding a replacement for increasingly ineffective antibiotics. The British Science Festival, in September 2015, heard from a microbial disease specialist who painted the possibility of an apocalyptic scenario in Britain if antibiotics fail.[26]

All that can be stated with any certainty is that the healthier and more aware the base population is, the better it will cope in future. Also, that proper planning and strategies for future health demands, pharmaceutical developments, and possible disasters, needs an NHS with firm financial clout. All possible resources – from contributory and insurance policies, pharmaceutical companies, charities and the state – must unite for this.

Embed the WTF test in everything

The trouble with monoliths is that they develop their own obscure language which in time becomes a vital form of self-protection and self-justification. A shield impenetrable by truth. I give you the NHS, the BBC, the Army, the Law, the Civil Service, local authorities: all of them bunkered happily in institutionalised obfuscation and acronym. My NHS, therefore, has simple semantics as one of its foundation stones. Language is primary; as much of a core component of any new health service as the desire to care for injured or sick people. If we cannot communicate, we are nothing.

We need to apply a WTF test from the top down. We need to imagine a blunt, streetwise Glaswegian asking 'Whit the f*** does that mean?' and then 'Why the f*** are we daein' this?' every single day. And, if there is no satisfactory answer, those in charge should go away and rethink. The WTF test is the first and best protocol of all.

There may already be a new breed running the NHS who write and speak simple English. I haven't heard their voice yet, because their impact will take ages to reach to the sharp end. We need change faster. Flabby, meaningless words are as much a signal of wasteful incompetence as urine bags which leak, computer systems which don't work, or truckloads of the wrong dressings. There is a fundamental symbolism in clear language. Let's begin there.

A health service (re)designed to help doctors give the best possible care to their patients

Mark Porter and Sally Al-Zaidy

A blank sheet of paper.

In order to restructure British healthcare for tomorrow – in any way – that is what you would need. A blank sheet of paper. But in reality there has never been, nor will there ever be, a blank sheet of paper for the NHS. Even in 1930 and 1938 when the BMA produced proposals for a national health service[1] [2] it was a case of bringing together what we already had, then adding to it, in order to make something better. Ten years later, Bevan established the NHS adopting many (though not all) of the BMA's key principles.[3]

There is much we would change about the NHS nearly 70 years on, but probably more that we would keep. Obvious though it sounds, perhaps the greatest thing the health service can offer the medical profession of tomorrow is the ability to give the best possible care to their patients. This essay will consider three ways in which an NHS for tomorrow would make this a reality.

First it will discuss the importance of maintaining and building upon the NHS's fundamental principles of equity, which allow doctors to focus on the clinical needs of their patients without worrying about ability to pay. Second it will consider how the NHS should be part of a much wider system designed to look after the whole person, not just disease. And third, it will consider what needs to be done to enable doctors and other clinicians to build clinical teams and partnerships across organisational boundaries and sectors, around the needs of their patients.

Maintain and improve equity

The founding and lasting principles of the NHS include that it should provide a comprehensive health service, free at the point of use and available to all on the basis of clinical need, not ability to pay. These fundamental principles of equity remain as important to the success of the NHS today as they did in 1948.

At its most basic level, equity represents the notion of fairness. From the egalitarian or social justice perspective – that most relevant to the NHS – three key assumptions underpin the debate. Healthcare is a right; resources for allocating healthcare are finite; and health policy should design fair or 'just' mechanisms for allocating them.[4] In this context equity 'refers to receiving treatment according to need and the financing of healthcare according to ability to pay'.[5]

The NHS seeks to achieve equity through the principles of universality and comprehensiveness, neither of which has a fixed definition.[6] Universality is multi-dimensional and encapsulates a statement of intent in relation to who can access the NHS, on what basis, and also a sense of sameness in terms of users' experience of the health service. Sameness could be interpreted in a number of ways including in relation to the quality, range, availability and/or effectiveness of services. Comprehensive refers to what services the NHS offers, which also encapsulates an element of sameness. However there is no explicit benefits package in the NHS.

The overarching method of achieving equity in the NHS is through it being funded by general taxation. Taxation in the UK is progressive overall, so the more you earn, the more you contribute. Further, funding healthcare through general taxation has been shown to be more equitable than other methods such as social health insurance.[7] Through its approach to financing therefore, the NHS achieves the highest possible level of equity.

Another key national level approach to ensure equity is the use of a resource allocation formula by which funds pooled centrally are allocated to regions in the country (i.e. commissioners). The NHS (in England) has used a weighted capitation formula for this purpose since the 1970s, devised by an independent body, the Advisory Committee on Resource Allocation (ACRA).

Finally a number of policies applied nationally in England seek to standardise users' experience of the health service, for example waiting time targets, the right to NICE (National Institute for Health and Care Excellence) -approved drugs and technologies and patient choice policies. For example, patients have had 'free choice' of any NHS or registered independent sector provider for routine elective care since 2008.

Most importantly, through funding collectively, the NHS offers the UK population financial protection from sudden high costs of healthcare at what may be a very vulnerable time. By comparison, in the US, which has a private health insurance-based system, medical debt is the largest cause of personal bankruptcy.[8] So by removing questions or concerns over ability to pay, doctors are able to focus solely on the clinical needs of their patients, eliminating what would otherwise be an unhelpful distraction in the doctor-patient relationship.

But the NHS' approach to equity is not perfect and improvements could be made. Our NHS for tomorrow would eliminate the most glaring, remaining circumstance under which ability to pay does determine access to healthcare services; prescription charges. User charges in general are both regressive and inequitable, as they limit access to healthcare on the basis of wealth. Prescription charges have been abolished in Scotland, Wales and Northern Ireland. The BMA continues to call for England to follow suit.

Standardisation mechanisms that ensure a degree of sameness in users' experience of the NHS have their drawbacks. For example, many patient choice policies in England promote a consumerist model in the NHS. Our NHS for tomorrow would focus on meaningful patient choice, decoupled from market mechanisms,[9] and based on more than just limited waiting time and misleading avoidable death[10] information. Politicians and policymakers would be more honest with the public about the extent to which choice can be delivered within the NHS, including in many cases the trade-off between short-term considerations, such as choice of provider, and long-term considerations, planned, sustainable NHS services.

In addition to their drawbacks, these standardisation mechanisms only go so far to ensure sameness in users' experience of the NHS. There is variation (albeit usually at the margins) in what constitutes a comprehensive health service depending on where you live. Priority setting at a CCG (clinical commissioning group) level takes the form of exclusion lists of specific treatments that are not available in that area. Treatments are designated as 'low-priority' either because they offer 'poor clinical value', such as surgery for lower back pain and grommets, or 'they are not clinically necessary', for example cosmetic surgery such as breast enlargement or reduction, or tattoo removal.[11] And eligibility criteria or thresholds, also decided at CCG level, set out which patients are eligible for referral or treatment on the NHS. Examples include score cards to qualify for hip and knee replacements, IVF and tonsillectomy.[12]

So how can this situation be improved? Centralise all decision making that determines access to services? Increase the NHS budget so that everyone really can have everything? Unfortunately, neither are particularly workable solutions. While unpalatable on many levels and from a number of viewpoints, including that of doctors,[13] such variation appears to be an inevitable consequence of devolving responsibility and funding away from the centre, to commissioners, in the context of scarcity of resources.

Our NHS for tomorrow would improve the quality, validity and robustness of the evidence base that underpins such decision-making. Something we know varies between commissioners,[14] with the Nuffield Trust having found 'priority setting in the NHS... to have more weaknesses than strengths'.[15] Efforts could be made at a national or regional level for these methods to be standardised and improved. The NHS should help its commissioners make more robust and equitable decisions that truly reflect the needs and values of their patient populations.[16]

Ultimately, variation should correspond with the specific needs of the patient population, as based upon sound population-level needs assessment, and within a robust social values framework. Using that developed by University College London and King's College London,[17] NHS commissioners need particular support on the 'process' elements of the framework, *how* decisions are made in terms of transparency, accountability and participation.[18]

But variation in users' experience of the NHS arises for other reasons too. The NHS Atlas of Variation in Healthcare highlights wide disparities in terms of the investment made, activity undertaken and outcomes achieved across the country[19] – disparities that cannot be justified on the basis of the differing needs of populations. Often the variance in the rates of intervention between different populations is in reality due to both demand and supply factors.[20] For example, where there are high rates of intervention, this does not necessarily translate to there being high levels of demand (such as severe need). It may be more a question of supply-led demand where provider capacity determines the rate of intervention[21] or alternatively path dependency where historic patterns of service delivery or resources determine them.[22]

Another reason for the varying levels of value in healthcare that the Atlas reveals, arises from an inconsistency in applying clinical research and best clinical practice. In 2011 the BMJ estimated that just 11% of the 3,000 treatments included in their clinical evidence handbook were 'known' to be clinically effective and a further 23% were only 'likely' to be beneficial. However it also estimated that 50% had unknown effectiveness.[23]

Our NHS for tomorrow would tackle variation by applying clinical research and best clinical practice more consistently. NICE should be liberated from the direction of the secretary of state. It would undertake a 'catch up' exercise to reduce the 'unknown effectiveness' category over time. And in the meantime, more attention would be paid to NICE's existing 'do not do' database, listing interventions that it advises against being used in the NHS, on the basis of lack of evidence on the benefits.[24]

But directing efforts solely at commissioners, as is the intention through the rollout of the RightCare programme to all CCGs,[25] will be insufficient. Providers need to take clinical governance as, if not more, seriously than financial governance. There should be greater investment in and commitment to the main components of clinical governance: risk management; clinical audit; education, training and continuing professional development; evidence-based care and effectiveness; patient and carer experience and involvement; and staffing and staff management. The focus on financial management in the NHS by the government and national regulators is too dominant. Our NHS for tomorrow would encourage hospitals and other providers to make clinical governance their core mission.

Beyond the medical model

The NHS is facing a number of challenges arising from the UK's ageing population and changing epidemiology. Higher prevalence of long-term conditions, multiple co-morbidities and people with complex needs is fuelling rising demand. Focusing on disease and its treatment, while sidelining ill-health prevention, as well as the sociocultural and psychological aspects of care and recovery will do little to meet these challenges. Medicalising all of society's problems will not work and thus the medical model as the central pillar of the health service can only go so far.

Our NHS for tomorrow would rebalance the health service to give equal priority to the promotion and maintenance of health, alongside the treatment of disease and injury. Others, including NHS England,[26] agree. In fact one of the BMA's key proposals for a national health service was that the medical system should be directed to positive health and the prevention of disease.[27]

However the current commissioning arrangements in England are too fragmented and limited in scope to achieve these aims. This is not only the product of the recent, major reorganisation of the health service through the Health and Social Care Act 2012, but also that of many layers and years of often conflicting health policies directed by successive governments.

Responsibility for health and public health were split between the NHS and local government (respectively) from the outset. Public health was brought into the NHS in 1974, then returned to local authorities in April 2013. This recent separation has put too much distance between public health expertise and NHS planning and service provision. All at a time when strong ill health prevention and population-level needs assessment should underpin the work of the NHS. Similarly, England, Scotland and Wales are still trying to make sense of the separation between health and social care, despite being embedded nearly 70 years ago when the NHS was established.

Various attempts to fix the system are underway, some with the potential to fragment the system further and all raising a multitude of structural and cultural challenges. National-level policies such as the better care fund in England and the Public Bodies (Joint Working) (Scotland) Act 2014 encourage the pooling of a portion of health and social care budgets. Regional devolution in England, such as in Greater Manchester, will see the full merging of health, public health and social care budgets and commissioning responsibility from April 2016. But what none of these policies do is address the longstanding issue around eligibility to receive free social care. The public must understand what they might be expected to pay for personal care now and in the future.[28] But in England the situation is getting worse with the delay of the cap on care costs from April 2016, to 2020.

Our NHS for tomorrow would follow a national framework for how NHS, public health and social care will be funded, commissioned and organised in the future, and in order to be fit to meet the future needs of the population. This would involve cross-party political consensus in order to ensure stability and certainty in the direction of travel. And it would sit alongside a realistic timeframe for implementation, for example over the course of the next two terms of government. Any national strategy would allow room for local areas to build upon existing arrangements that are working well.[29]

But even with NHS, public health and social care services brought closer together, this can only do so much to improve the population's health.

The most recent estimate suggests that healthcare only contributes 25% towards overall health. Socio-economic factors such as housing, employment and education contribute 50%, environmental factors 10% and genetics 15%.[30]

Despite the range of actions put forward in the Marmot Review to reduce health inequalities, there are signs that inequalities have continued to widen[31] [32] [33] and BMA members have expressed concern that this will be worsened by recent austerity measures and welfare reform.[34] Of particular concern is the disproportionate burden on vulnerable and disadvantaged groups (such as unemployed, disabled, and elderly people), as well as on children and families. The impact of austerity measures and welfare reform – combined with a period of persistent increases in the general price level of goods, services and rent – has been to move more people away from achieving a minimum income for healthy living.[35] There is a clear concern that those parts of the UK more heavily reliant on public sector employment will be disproportionately affected by austerity measures. For example, the public sector accounts for over a quarter of employment in Northern Ireland, nearly a quarter of employment in Wales, and more than one in five jobs in Scotland and the North East.[36]

Our NHS for tomorrow would be part of a wider system working nationally, regionally and locally to address the social determinants of health. Nationally, UK governments would mandate a 'health in all policies' approach to ensure that health is incorporated into all of their decision-making areas. The success of this approach can be found in various countries, including in Finland in relation to child and adolescent health.[37] Regionally, all planning and delivery of public services would come much closer together (as part of the national framework mentioned above) ensuring that policies and actions are joined up in the pursuit of population health improvement. Locally, doctors would be able to offer patients access to non-medical support in the community, helping to alleviate some of the social determinants of ill health.

These measures combined would help doctors treat the whole person, not just disease, and be confident that the system is designed to pre-empt, pick up and address patients' and society's much wider needs: those that go far beyond the reach of the medical model.

Integration and coordination, not competition

There is growing recognition and consensus that the NHS needs to work differently, around the changing needs of the population, and through greater provider integration. Yet alongside this there has been a frustrating lack of recognition that the national, legislative and regulatory frameworks in place are actively working against this goal.

In England, there is now a major discord between the renewed emphasis on provider integration and collaboration in national-level policy and the legislation that underpins how the health service is run. The NHS does not operate as a full-blown market, but numerous policies around choice and competition seek to create quasi- or internal market conditions. The introduction of the purchaser-provider split in 1991 was followed by further reforms in the 2000s, introducing greater plurality of provision through the national procurement of ISTCs, choice of provider policies and the national tariff. The Health and Social Care Act 2012 then embedded market mechanisms into the NHS further, such as through the concurrent duties of Monitor and the Competition and Markets Authority in relation to anti-competitive behaviour, as well as the requirement for CCGs to either competitively tender or put services out to 'any qualified provider' for the majority of their contracts.

Yet there is little or no evidence to support the internal market or market competition.[38] Evidence from both the NHS[39] [40] and internationally[41] shows marketisation to incur new costs. And there is no conclusive evidence to suggest that the private or commercial sector offers improved services or better value for money in return.[42]

The current frameworks also act as a major barrier to more provider integration and greater cooperation and coordination between services. Doctors cannot and do not work in isolation, with the concept of the clinical team within a hospital ward or GP practice being well established. However it is the extended clinical team, made up of clinicians and other professionals across different organizations and sectors that doctors are struggling to build. And as is the case with commissioning in England, service provision has become incredibly fragmented.

There are no plans to address this discord between national-level policy and legislation through regulatory change. While the Five Year Forward View vanguard sites will receive dedicated support to understand how to navigate the situation, it is unlikely that new models of care will spread across England more widely, at pace and at scale as intended, if no national action is taken.

However the NHS can and does operate without the internal market. Scotland and Wales have long since abolished the purchaser-provider split. While technically Northern Ireland has retained it, no further market-based policies have been added and it operates a system largely based on consultation and co-operation.[43]

Our NHS for tomorrow would abolish the purchaser provider split in England. The least disruptive route to achieve this aim would be to re-establish commissioning as a strategic planning function, and separate it from purchasing by removing other market mechanisms. Duties to prevent anticompetitive behaviour in the NHS, currently held by Monitor and the Competition and Markets Authority, would go. And CCGs would have the autonomy to choose the most appropriate procurement processes for the services that they wish to put in place for their patient populations.[44]

Strategic planning should continue to be led by clinicians, but with wider input from across the profession, particularly other sectors such as secondary care and public health. The process of planning and provision would be led by the public sector and there would be a genuine partnership approach between commissioners and providers.

Integration and coordination would be the driving force behind the NHS in the future. Patients and service users would not encounter barriers, gaps or 'bumps' when moving around the health system and between different providers of their care. Providers of healthcare would have access to up-to-date patient information in order that they do not unwittingly create any such discontinuities. Commissioners would work to ensure that patients experience cohesive and responsive care by putting in place integrated care pathways for particular patient groups, and by working with healthcare providers to ensure they understand their role and responsibilities as part of an integrated pathway of care.

Around 6% of NHS services were delivered by the independent sector in 2014/15, amounting to £6.9 billion of NHS funding.[45] This includes general and acute, accident and emergency, community health, maternity, mental health and learning disability services. Yet we know very little about whether independent sector provision of NHS services adds much or any value to patients. Nor do we know (and nor do some seem to care) how it affects local NHS providers.

Independent sector provision has and will continue to destabilise NHS providers by breaking up existing services, with the more profitable elements being the ones most successfully contracted out. An independent impact assessment in Coastal West Sussex found that a proposed multi-year contract for musculoskeletal services, if placed with an independent sector provider, would have made the existing provider, an NHS foundation trust, both financially and clinically unviable within five years.[46] An independent service review in Nottingham found that the transfer of outpatient dermatology services to an ISTC (independent sector treatment centre) led to a 'near collapse of acute and paediatric dermatology services' within the local NHS acute trust and local health economy more generally.[47]

Our NHS for tomorrow would promote a publicly-funded and publicly-provided health system, with the underlying principle that the NHS is the preferred provider. It would value a long-term strategy to secure the future of the NHS for the benefit of patients, over short-sighted or short-term goals for the benefit of markets and political ideology.

Conclusion

This essay has outlined three ways in which the BMA would redesign the NHS in order to help doctors of tomorrow give the best possible care to their patients.

The NHS's fundamental principles of equity would be maintained and improved upon, allowing doctors to continue to treat patients purely on the basis of their clinical needs, not ability to pay. Prescription charges would be abolished in England as they have been elsewhere in the UK. Patient choice policies, which in part seeks to standardise users' experience of the NHS, would be made more meaningful by decoupling them from market mechanisms. The quality of priority setting in the NHS would be improved to truly reflect both the needs and values of communities. And variation that cannot be justified by the differing needs of populations would be tackled through a more consistent application of clinical research and best clinical practice, as well as by clinical governance becoming the core mission of providers of NHS care.

Next, our NHS for tomorrow would help doctors move beyond the medical model by operating within a much wider system designed to address the social determinants of health. Equal priority would be given to the promotion and maintenance of health, alongside the treatment of disease and injury. A national framework for how NHS, public health and social care will come together in the future would build upon arrangements already working well locally. A 'health in all policies' approach would be mandated by UK governments. This would be reinforced regionally, ensuring that policies and actions are joined up in the pursuit of population health improvement, as well as locally, by doctors being able to offer patients access to non-medical support in the community.

Lastly, doctors would be enabled to build clinical teams and partnerships across organisational boundaries and sectors, around the needs of their patients. Integration and coordination would be the driving force behind the NHS. To achieve this the purchaser-provider split would be abolished in England as it has been in Scotland and Wales. Commissioning would be re-established as a strategic planning function, by separating it from purchasing and removing other market mechanisms. Duties to prevent anticompetitive behaviour in the NHS, currently held by Monitor and the Competition and Markets Authority, would go. And CCGs would be able to decide what procurement processes to use to secure services. The long-term sustainability of the NHS would always trump the pursuit of the internal market and the use of independent sector providers. Because where would we all be if the NHS slowly disintegrated, whether by specific design or unintended consequence?

Our NHS for tomorrow would, fundamentally, be built around the needs of people. Treating them as patients where appropriate, but within an integrated system that recognises the central importance of care organised around people's needs, in pursuit of the fullest definition of healthcare – a state of complete physical, mental and social well-being and not merely the absence of disease or infirmity.

It is something wonderful that our society has reached the point where the choice to do this lies within our reach, and depends only on our decision to do so.

On the brink of disruption: how can universal healthcare make the most of radical innovation?

Steve Melton

Kodak and the curse of the incumbent

In the 1970s, Steven J Sasson, an electrical engineer at Kodak, approached his management team and presented a radical new idea: the digital camera. At the time, home computing was still in its infancy, let alone tablets, digital devices or cameras. Old-school film dominated photography, and represented the vast majority of Kodak's business. Recalling his presentation, Sasson later said: 'It was filmless photography. So management's reaction was, "that's cute – but don't tell anyone about it."'[1]

The rest is history. Now, digital cameras not only dominate photography sales, but smartphones prevail on the streets, laptops link corners of the globe, and GoPros follow astronauts into space. Digital cameras changed the entire digital and communication landscape. But even as digital cameras started to emerge, and began their march to dominance, Kodak stuck firmly to film. They missed their moment. They were too successful selling film to see a challenge, and could not see the long-term change digital technology ushered in. In the end, Kodak declared bankruptcy in 2012. In the same year, £568 million worth of digital cameras were sold in the UK alone.[2]

Time and again, in all industries, we see this pattern: the curse of the incumbent. Organisations that do well out of an existing market or system tend not to be very good at reinventing it. The skills they needed to make it in the first place are usually different to the skills needed to adapt. They have little incentive to pursue radical ideas, on both a financial and emotional level: it often looks like supporting a new technology would cannibalise their existing business, and human nature errs towards loss aversion, rather than preferring to seek potential gain.

So most organisations are happy to carry on doing the same thing, and if they are already successful, the instinct for institutional conservatism can be overpowering. Even if most do not have the spectacular misjudgement of Kodak, they tend to see new developments as risks rather than opportunities, and be far slower-moving than newer, more agile organisations.

Healthcare on the brink of disruption

Kodak's example has lessons for any industry. But it is particularly relevant to healthcare today - and if we want to guarantee universal healthcare for tomorrow, understanding this dynamic is essential. To explain why, it is worth thinking about some of the recent advances in healthcare.

Technology

Since 1987, the number of beds in the NHS has approximately halved.[3] It would be easy to mistake this for rationing: it is really a function of increased efficiency. Thirty years ago, a common elective surgical procedure – a knee arthroscopy, for example, where the knee is examined and repaired – would have involved around 2-3 days in hospital, and a procedure in an operating theatre that lasted around two hours.

Now, the vast majority of arthroscopies are carried out within a single day, in about an hour, with a laparoscopic procedure (keyhole surgery). As a result, the patient does not need to stay overnight, the surgery is less invasive and less risky – and the NHS saves money by avoiding the need to pay for a bed, nursing and overnight care.

This pattern is repeated in almost every specialty, and represents considerable improvements on healthcare even five or 10 years ago. But they pale in comparison to the radical technologies that will mature in the coming decades. The technology emerging today makes science fiction look backward. Biological 3D printing recently became a reality when a team at Princeton printed a bionic ear.[4] Thumbnail-sized medical tattoos allow us to monitor sun exposure, heart rate, temperature, oxygen levels. EU-funded researchers have developed a 'brain-neural-computer interface' which enables a human to control an exoskeleton with their mind.

New models possible

As the technology grows, so does the potential for new ways of delivering care.

Circle, the company I lead, recently started a teledermatology service. GPs can take hi-res imagery of skin conditions and send them to a specialist consultant. The system means that malignant or troubling skin conditions can be quickly filtered out from the majority of benign issues – and hospital care or surgery reserved for only those who need it. It uses one specialist image device, a dermatoscope, attached to a near-ubiquitous consumer technology: an iPhone.

With this new system, we have found that approximately 60% of patients do not need a consultant appointment, but have a benign condition the GP can look after. Waiting times were previously 16 weeks for non-cancer skin conditions; they can receive a teledermatology opinion within 48 hours. This is both better for the patient, and significantly better value for the NHS.

Examples like our service will only grow. In time, many of the buzzwords we hear flying around – self-care, app care, tele-health and the automated self – will become living realities. Crucially, many of these advances will not come from the UK, Europe, or the West. Some of the most innovative approaches are emerging in the developing world. Devi Shetty's approach to cardiac surgery in India is well known; perhaps less well known is that on the other side of the continent, Apollo Hospitals is pioneering robotic surgery.

Demographic change

Just as technology is set to transform our society, so is demographic change. On current trends, and failing some unforeseen massive social change, Britain will have 20 million people over the age of 65 by 2031.[5] With it, healthcare demand will inexorably increase.

These future patients are more likely than any generation yet to be active consumers, rather than passive recipients, of their care. They are used to making informed choices in most aspects of their lives, from homes to holidays. Healthcare, in time, will be no different.

Combined with the potential for technology to free up information to consumers, then the coming of an ageing society is not just a simple increase in demand: it will also bring a radically different sort of customer to health. It will be the 'consumerisation' of health.

The NHS as an incumbent

In short, we are on the cusp of a revolution, in what technology can achieve, what models of care are possible, in overall demand and in patients' expectations. Few revolutions are bloodless, though. The question is whether universal healthcare as we currently know it is capable of adapting.

On the face of it, today's NHS has the potential to be a classic incumbent. It is often a monopoly provider, especially in some areas experiencing particularly fast changes, such as acute and primary care. It is, naturally, focussed on being the best it can be. It has vast organisational experience, built over decades, on how to run services – as we currently understand them. It has a large managerial superstructure ensuring the smooth operation of services – as we currently understand them.

In short, the NHS risks being the classic sort of organisation that fails to champion change, even if it would benefit in the long term – simply because it is so focussed on what it does now. The point about the incumbents' curse is that even the highest-performing organisations risk missing the chance to change, or seeing a radical new way of doings things. It is precisely success that can prevent rapid change.

What the NHS has unquestionably provided is equitable access, and a sense of fairness in how healthcare resources are allocated. Polling is generally clear that the NHS is popular. So Kodak's example raises a question. We currently have a healthcare system that is generally popular, free at the point of use, and largely organised by a single organisation - but facing an exceptionally volatile period, led by demographic change and technology.

So is it possible for the NHS to break free of the incumbents' curse? Given the scale and pace of change, what sort of policies, structure and culture will take advantage of the brave new world – and which would mean the end of universal healthcare?

What is the answer to harnessing disruption, rather than being destroyed by it? To me, this is the key question when considering universal healthcare for tomorrow. The rest of this essay will seek to answer what the answer might be.

Avoid the macro

My answer is that first, we should not get too obsessed with system-wide structures. The classic response to questions over the NHS's future is to reach for institutional reorganisation. There is a good reason for this: this represents the clearest powers vested in secretaries of state for health. Politicians naturally reach for the most obvious levers of power, which are either passing laws or regulations, or reshuffling the organisations that manage the NHS.

In recent years, there has also been a push to weed out poor performance with a range of central incentives and penalties. The trend in the past 24 months has been towards the latter, with a range of personal and professional sanctions for underperformance. Both approaches – to reorganise the system and to punish individuals – are useful politically, giving a sense of energy and acting in patients' interests.

They also entirely misunderstand the nature of a large system like the NHS. The NHS already has intelligent people with a strong vocational drive. Simply pushing them harder does not work. Reorganising the system might bring marginal benefits, but almost all reorganisations overestimate the eventual gain, and underestimate the effect of uncertainty and job churn as the new structure settles in. The usual and obvious route – restructuring and downward pressure – is not, in other words, going to be enough.

Payment systems

Similarly, we should not get too obsessed with payment systems. As the leader of a private healthcare organisation, people often assume that I would prefer an insurance-funded model in the UK – or an entirely privatised free market. But then as a company that provides services to the NHS, other people also often assume that deep down, we quite like a state-organised service funded through general taxation.

I tend to frustrate both groups, by saying that endlessly discussing payment mechanisms tends to be a red herring. Most developed countries have healthcare systems that offer good access to healthcare with reasonable outcomes. A mixed model of state and private provision and funding is common across the developed world, and only the USA is a real outlier in poor outcomes, access and value.

This range of models shows there is no single answer: no magic formula that combines individual, employer or state funding, or state, private and voluntary provision. Indeed, the range of models suggests that we should see healthcare funding as a function of political economy. Few countries decided in the abstract what sort of system they wanted – most developed theirs in a manner that reflects their politics, economics and social expectations. None operate in a vacuum. None have found the perfect answer.

Some debate on payment structure is natural, of course – but in searching for the recipe that will mean future universal healthcare succeeds or fails, it is not, in my view, the crucial ingredient.

Funding

The same goes for funding. A slightly facile debate surrounds healthcare funding in the UK. Commentators on the left can regularly be heard talking about the 'underfunding' of the NHS, and bemoaning cuts to healthcare. On the right, meanwhile, accusations of waste, over-staffing with managers, fat paychecks for NHS leaders and inefficiency abound.

In fact, in total the UK spends slightly below the OECD average on healthcare (8.4% of GDP compared to 8.8% average)[6], but 83% of that is state spending – which is one of the highest proportions in the OECD. So most other countries spend more, but the difference is made up by consumers, with co-payments or insurance payments. In other words, the UK government is neither absurdly generous, nor radically under-funding the system.

The UK is different in one sense. Assuming no radical changes in politics, health spending will continue to rise up to 2020. At the same time, other areas of state spending have been reduced. Again, assuming no radical changes to government policy, they will face further reductions. Healthcare commentators have an unfortunate tendency to see no further than the borders of the NHS: looking at state health spending in the context of what other areas are getting would perhaps be enlightening, and a better basis for thinking about how much we under- or over-fund the NHS. Anyone thinking that it is harshly under-funded should perhaps talk to a lawyer about legal aid: and should perhaps consider the state has functions outside health, and if money is tight, state spending becomes a zero-sum game.

Yet even with that in mind, more funding does not add up to creating universal healthcare for the future: for the simple reason that funding is always relative to population needs. Current demographic trends are unremitting. It is almost – almost – pointless to say the NHS needs more money, because it is always going to need more if it is to meet future demand with the current system. Arguing for an increase in funding is Sisyphean policy. Alone, it might offer short-term relief: but it will not guarantee universal healthcare for the future.

A culture of innovation

If not payment structure, and not funding, then what? My answer is primarily, about culture – and specifically, a culture of innovation. The incumbents' curse shows that organisations with a vested interest in one system are generally bad at adapting to a new one. Healthcare, on the brink of a revolution in technology, new models, demographics and patient expectations, and with a single dominant provider like the NHS, fits that category.

As such, I believe that to create universal healthcare for tomorrow we need to focus on how to create innovation at pace and scale. Ideas matter, and the main task is to understand how we help new ideas spread and grow. There are four things that need to happen: developing a better attitude to risk; greater diversity; thinking about integrated models; and clinical engagement.

A better attitude to risk

Silicon Valley attracts praise and mockery in equal measure: its companies are seen as both world-changing and spectacularly hubristic. Its real success, however, lies in creating an environment that allows sensible risk-taking. An entrepreneur on the west coast of America will assume that you will fail several times before succeeding. Failure is seen as inevitable in a fast-changing world: what matters is how quickly failure is learnt from, and then translated into a future success. Risk-taking, within reason, is seen as a natural part of working life.

Medicine is, in some senses, right to retain a degree of caution. People's lives are at stake and most patients simply want good care. Taking risks is not an end in itself. But, too often, healthcare management in the NHS steers for the known and familiar by default, or even attempts to avoid risk altogether. This is to misunderstand the nature of progress. The reason the entrepreneurs' mantra of 'fail fast and fail better' works is that it is far from being a tech-utopian dream, it is actually a very practical method. It recognises that doing things differently is difficult, and that mistakes are likely, and that it is better to learn from mistakes than try to avoid them altogether. It is, for all its zeal, a very down-to-earth way of incubating successful ideas.

If the NHS is to survive the incumbents' curse, it needs to learn from this culture.

A better attitude to risk could be achieved a number of ways: there are legal protections, for example, that could be introduced for leaders who try new approaches (at present they are often liable if they vary from normal practice). Leaders who create new ideas could receive more formal support from the centre, whether rhetorical or financial. Funding already exists for transformation projects: similar funding streams could be attached more specifically to radical innovations, or changed into prizes or seed-funding to attract creative ideas.

Really, though, this is a question of leadership from the top. Political and NHS leaders need to be unequivocal to managers elsewhere in the system: you have a licence to innovate, and we will support you in taking sensible risks, and trying new things.

Diversity

One of the reasons incumbents fail is that they inadvertently attract people like themselves. They become successful in an industry, and their recruitment starts to become self-selecting. They both hire people who fit the mould, and people who fit the mould find them attractive. In time, this can create monocultures: collections of people who are, in most respects, exactly like each other. Unsurprisingly, this tends to create one-dimensional thinking.

In innovative organisations, the opposite is true. There is diversity, in every sense – in thinking styles, personalities, backgrounds and approaches. There is a well-studied trend in the impact of immigrants on economies: roughly a third of US-based Nobel prizes in the 20th century were to immigrants to the USA,[7] while famous companies like Google, eBay, Goldman Sachs, Yahoo!, Colgate, Pfizer, Procter & Gamble were all founded by immigrants. Circle, for its part, was founded by a doctor and a banker who came to the UK from Iran. Outsiders tend to come up with new ways of looking at problems: organisations that innovate see creativity in difference, and encourage challenge from within.

In a complex system like the NHS, diversity has a number of meanings. The usual sense of diversity – racial, gender and social diversity – is crucial, and the NHS has taken a number of steps to advance on this front. But it also means being open to new types of organisation. The NHS has always used the private sector, with a particular gathering of pace under Labour from 2001 onwards. Under the Coalition, there was new excitement about the voluntary sector, and use of employee-owned and mutual organisations 'spinning out' of the public sector.

Yet there is still a reticence about explicitly saying the NHS wants to access the best ideas: there is a hesitancy and fear about being seen to 'privatise' or 'profiteer'. Even non-profit social enterprises – or co-owned companies like Circle, where staff are also shareholders – have their motives questioned. This is not sustainable, if the NHS wants to harness innovation. Just as individual diversity adds to the richness of any single organisation, a diverse range of organisations adds to the overall ability of a system to adapt.

A common way for large companies to avoid the incumbents' curse, for example, is to snap up new innovators. Google or Microsoft or Facebook take stakes in start-ups doing interesting things. They do this to access the people or intellectual property of the new startup – and to ingest it into their existing operations. The NHS will perhaps never act so aggressively, but the principle is the same. It should be scanning the world for the best ideas and innovations, and be completely agnostic about where they come from.

Government policy needs to be equally clear: diversity is good, and that means a fearless search for the innovators, whether they are in the public, private, voluntary or social enterprise sector. When they are found, they need to be encouraged into the NHS.

Integrated models

The third feature is to think about opportunities across organisations. Healthcare is currently structured into silos. GPs, hospitals, community providers and social care are distinct organisations, formally tasked with individually pursuing one aspect of care.

This has a number of effects. It means that organisations tend to protect their own finances, rather than seek a system-wide view. There has been a notable trend, for example, in the past two years for commissioners to seek budget surpluses, at the expense of providers. At the same time, some bodies have seen expanded budgets – notably inspectors and central regulators – while others have reduced. Some hospitals have income from a range of specialist and teaching services, while others (particularly smaller hospitals) have a far narrower income stream, and are much more vulnerable to policy changes.

If we spent as much time looking at under- or over-resourcing within the NHS as we did discussing its overall funding, that would be significantly more helpful. The disjointed nature of healthcare makes that difficult. It also means that in an age of financial pressures, it is difficult to achieve further efficiencies. Most individual organisations within the NHS will struggle to balance the books on their own; but there might be opportunities to make systems as a whole more efficient. For example, an average acute hospital with a large deficit will, after a number of years of efficiency drives, struggle to make really significant progress. But seen in the context of its surrounding system – where there could be opportunities to keep patients out of hospital in cheaper settings closer to home, or to improve links with social care to speed up their transfer out of hospital – the efficiency challenge may be more manageable.

The same goes for innovations. The best ideas will come from thinking about entire disease areas or populations in the round, rather than just looking at individual organisations. To take one example, for the past two years, Circle has been running an integrated contract for MSK services in Bedfordshire. We take a previously disjointed set of services, and unite them into a single service. Where previously, a patient would have bounced between GPs and hospital and community services, we now offer them specialist triage – meaning they are far more likely to see the right clinician first time round. Because we are managing the entire system, we can track a host of outcomes for the first time – and hold providers to account for the care they offer. All of this is for a capped budget covering the entire population, which is less than the Commissioner was projected to spend.

In other words, we offer better care for less spending. It is exactly the sort of innovation the NHS needs, and it is only possible by thinking about healthcare systems in an integrated fashion. To give credit where it is due, this is the direction of the NHS under Simon Stevens' Five Year Forward View. Policy needs to be backed up with moral support too. Our experience in Bedford is that it does not take structural change – tinkering or reorganising – but a mindset. Circle's Bedfordshire contract did not require new laws or reorganisations: it took commissioners with imagination and determination. This sort of thinking at a system-wide, integrated level, is essential to adapting to the fast-changing healthcare landscape.

Clinical engagement

The final element is clinical engagement. Most service companies allow professionals to rise into leadership positions, and their business is based on tapping the expertise and ideas of skilled workers. Think about a law, accountancy or management consultancy: their main product is the experience and training of their staff, and after a few decades' service their staff can often expect to become partners.

This has a number of benefits. It means that the front-line service is well-connected to management. Leaders understand the core service, and have the credibility to talk about and shape their organisation. Most importantly, it encourages innovation – as the people who are best-placed to spot new ideas are active participants in their employers.

Healthcare, however, has traditionally been run on different lines. In many hospitals there is a sharp divide between clinicians and managers. Relatively few clinicians end up leading hospitals, either because they believe they should not enter leadership roles, or want to but lack the support and training to make the step up. Every hospital has a medical director, but the very fact a specific role is created points to the traditional gap – try to imagine a law firm that delegated responsibility for law to a single 'head of legal' partner.

This in turn feeds a culture which is usually hierarchical. Most hospitals and health systems are shaped like pyramids, where orders are sent down and up a chain of command. Delegation is common, but true responsibility and devolved accountability are rare. Ask a nurse on an average ward about their ability to make everyday decisions about the hospital, and other than individual patients' care, the answer will too often involve some sense of ambitions stifled by bureaucracy.

This is one root cause of poor morale in the NHS. It is also an appalling waste of the commitment of NHS staff. Any organisations' best chance of reinventing itself – of staying ahead of new trends – is the experience and enthusiasm of its front-line people. If we want universal healthcare, then we need this to change. To be clear, there are some hospitals where clinicians have assumed leadership positions, and some excellent hospitals which engage their staff. On the whole, though, good clinical engagement remains an unfortunate exception.

Circle's model is different. It is explicitly based on clinical engagement, and allying clinical and non-clinical backgrounds in management. I come from a retail background, for example; our hospitals are led by physios, nurses and professional managers; we have surgeons leading business development and people from manufacturing running health systems; each hospitals' board is majority-clinician.

Within hospitals, we form Clinical Units of no more than 100 staff led by a doctor, nurse and manager. At their most autonomous, these units manage their own budgets and make decisions about how to improve clinical outcomes and patient experience. Some units, at an earlier stage of their growth, have closer direction from the centre. The emphasis, though, is on frontline staff feeling it is within their power to change things for their patients.

The results are seen across our hospitals. When we took on a treatment centre in Nottingham, we saw a 20% increase in productivity compared to the previous operation – by asking staff to come up with creative solutions to improve care. When we ran Hinchingbrooke, an NHS acute hospital, over 1200 staff helped write a shared business plan – arguably one of the largest exercises in workplace democracy ever undertaken in UK health. When we choose a new clinical chair for our private hospitals, we asked the clinicians to ratify the decision. Our hospital design reflects staff input, from simple things like the fact our corridors are wider (because our porters said most hospitals' weren't wide enough) to a bespoke kitchen for our chefs, to a system where doctors are sent patients' photos and name – because our front-of-house team realized that shouting out names across a waiting room was very impersonal – to the fact our largest hospital doesn't have departments but lettered Gateways (as in Gateway A, B, C) so that other patients didn't know what procedure they needed. Our most important safety system allows any team member (not just a surgeon) to stop an operation if they feel something is wrong: a radical inversion of traditional power structures in hospitals.

These are only a few examples, and I certainly don't pretend that Circle has got everything right – and making sure staff feel they can contribute is a constant task, and a culture we constantly need to encourage. But these are small innovations that add up to a different way of doing things, and they rely on frontline staff feeling engaged. If the big challenge facing the NHS is taking advantage of new ideas, then clinical engagement is essential.

Conclusion

If the question, then, is how do we guarantee universal healthcare for tomorrow, then the answer can be found in looking at the Kodaks of this world: the organisations that fell to the incumbents' curse, that couldn't see the future because they were too heavily invested in the status quo.

We have to understand how to make the most of this dynamic. The answer isn't to be found in structure, and endless tinkering with payment mechanisms, or debating insurance or tax or public or private. The answer isn't to be found simply in funding, and pumping more (or less) money into healthcare. The answer is in the culture our health system promotes.

If we can create a healthcare system that rewards sensible risk-taking, that seeks true diversity, that thinks in an integrated way and that emphasises clinical engagement, then universal healthcare in this country is possible – and even has a bright future.

Turning healthcare on its head: the bidet revolution

Phil Hammond

'Why treat people and send them back to the conditions that make them sick?'

Michael Marmot

Universal healthcare in a society that is poor at prevention and in denial about death is like attempting to rescue a never ending stream of people from a river of illness. As science advances, we dive deeper and deeper into the river to pull out people who are sicker and sicker. The right to healthcare for all means that all too often, we treat the untreatable. Just because we can do something doesn't mean it's kind or wise to do so. A high-tech death can be very unkind. We spend so much time, effort and money pulling bodies to the riverbank, that we have no energy left to wander upstream and stop them falling in.

We live in a very unequal society, with huge disparities in both life expectancy and years lived in good health. Unless we can improve living and working conditions as well as lifestyle, with a strong emphasis on helping people to build resilience and stay mentally healthy, then no system of universal healthcare can cope, no matter how it is designed or funded. Those of us who are lucky enough to be healthy at present have a responsibility to try to remain so for as long as we can. The best hope for the NHS lies outside its structures. We must reduce poverty, promote healthy minds as well as bodies, lessen the burden of avoidable illness and permit choice in dying. There's more than enough unavoidable illness to keep the NHS in business.

This burden of avoidable illness could be further reduced by being honest about medical harm and the limits of medicine, and restricting over-medicalisation. Too many serious errors have been covered up and repeated in healthcare systems primed to protect professional, institutional, corporate and political reputations. Too many tests and treatments of marginal benefit turn healthy people into anxious patients. Enough people fall into the river of illness without being sucked in by the health industry.

There simply isn't a sound evidence base for the mass medication of the elderly, many of whom are either unable or unwilling to take so many drugs as prescribed. Waste due to ineffective treatments, non-attendance and non-adherence is significant. When patients are given the time and opportunity to fully understand and participate in decisions about their care, taking in the likely long-term risks and benefits in absolute as well as relative terms, they often choose less medicine, not more. Universal healthcare must also be prudent healthcare, using the minimal effective intervention wherever possible. Sound evidence based on real life data, as well as compassion, must inform health policy and provision.

Above all we must see healthcare in the context of all care. The boundaries between self, health and social care are entirely superficial, and we must extend our circles of collaboration and compassion as widely as possible and consider the environmental impact of what we do. Indigenous populations have a better understanding of how to live on this planet without taking so much as to threaten the health of future generations, and how to die. We only die once, and a gentle death for as many people as possible is the kindest service society can offer. As the Australian Aboriginal elder Dr Noel Nannup explains: 'Human beings are the carers of everything.' But to care for everything, we must first care for ourselves and build our own resilience. The NHS has had enough top down 're-disorganisations'. It's time for a bidet revolution. From the bottom up.

Healthcare begins with self-care

'Tell me, what is it you plan to do with your one wild and precious life?'

Mary Oliver

Self-care requires time to reflect and to do some 'self-work'. What are our goals, values, passions and purpose? Can we get near them without burning out? How can we be kind to our minds? How will we cope with pressure, failure, and adversity? Is our current lifestyle making avoidable disease more likely or even inevitable? Physical health stems from mental health, and learning how to be happy, how to self-care and how to cope under pressure should be taught and revisited at every stage of our lives. And we need to build happy and resilient cities, communities and organizations that promote mental health and allow individuals to flourish.

And yet as a society, we aren't great at talking about what matters most (mental health, sexual health, how we want to die). Self-care needs the self-knowledge that comes from these difficult conversations, and also self-love. Can you disappear inside your mind and like what you find there? Enjoying our own company is key to happiness and resilience. Accepting responsibility for self-care is also fundamental to the sustainability of universal healthcare. Every day we don't need to use the NHS, someone who does benefits.

The CLANGERS self-care model

Universal healthcare must embrace the continuum of self-care to intensive care, and I would restructure it around the CLANGERS model. The Clangers of the children's television series were, and probably still are, a community of mauve mice who spoke in whistles and ate sensible portions of soup, made by a dragon, and blue-string pudding, none of which was processed. They lived a simple yet serene life built around friendship, collaboration and enjoying the little things. Very seldom, if ever, did they need to go to hospital or indeed die, because they were so good at self-care and pleasuring themselves in a safe and sustainable way.

The Clangers' habit for a satisfying and meaningful life can be learned by anyone, at any age:

- *Connect* with the world around you. Reach out to people, pets, plants and places. We like to feel as if we belong, as part of something bigger. These connections are the cornerstones of your life. Take time and care to nurture them. And don't forget to connect with yourself.

- *Learn.* A purpose in life often stems from learning what matters most to you, developing a passion for learning and keeping your curiosity alive. Why do you get out of bed in the morning?

- *Be Active,* in mind and body. Rediscover activities and passions you left behind, and have the courage to try new ones. Aim for five portions of fun a day, each different, at least one outdoors and one that involves getting pleasantly breathless.

- *Notice,* and be present in, the world around you. Fill up your senses. Catch sight of the beautiful. Remark on the unusual. Enjoy the everyday. Savour the moment, and your place in it.

- *Give back.* Helping and caring for friends, strangers and those less fortunate than ourselves is fundamental to good emotional health. It cements us as part of a community and develops more meaningful connections and insights. The joy of being human is to be humane.

- *Eat well.* Learn what's good and enjoyable to eat, and in what quantities. Learn how to grow it, where to buy it and how to prepare it. Set time aside to sit and eat with friends and family.

- *Relax.* Take time to rest and reflect on the day you've had, reliving and re-savouring the happy memories and having gratitude for friends and family. Learn to meditate. Be kind to your mind and let it wind down and de-clutter.

- *Sleep.* Don't cheat on your sleep. It's vital recovery time for mind and body. Relaxing and winding down beforehand is key. Learning to housekeep your mind and deal with stress is vital.

Some lucky people will do all eight steps intuitively, partly out of habit. Others will struggle through sickness and circumstance but with support and time, can continuously improve and slowly raise their own bar – hopefully without the stress of comparing themselves to others. Your Clangers may be very different to my Clangers, the only rule is that we should try not to harm ourselves or others.

The 'clang' in CLANGERS comes from the government-funded Foresight report, 'Mental capital and wellbeing: making the most of ourselves in the 21st century'. It gathered the evidence on simple ways to a fulfilling life that just about anyone can do, irrespective of wealth or health. I added the 'ers' because they're also fundamental to living well and slowing down the rust. The CLANGERS model has not been widely tested in humans, although since it was published, it is being incorporated into a peer group-based intervention to improve health and wellbeing of parents and carers of disabled children. And a comprehensive school in Bridgend has adopted it as its banner for teaching health literacy.

CLANGERS in a healthcare setting

CLANGERS works not just as a model for living well, but also as a way of coping in adversity. When I interviewed patients and carers for a book about how to get the best from the NHS, it was striking how it fitted in with a successful model of patient engagement.

- *Connect* with the team treating you, and get to know them if you can. Know their names and something about them. It's easier to ask questions when you know someone.

- *Learn* as much as you can about your illness, the treatment options, what you are entitled to, the standards of care you should be getting, what you can do to improve your odds and who to speak to if you have concerns.

- *Be Active,* both in the management of your illness and preventing further illness, be your own advocate when you can, have others to act for you when you can't. The five portions of fun a day may be different to the ones you might enjoy when you're well, but still try to have the energy for joy, warmth and purpose each day.

- *Notice* the good and bad in your care, and speak up if you have any questions or concerns. Notice the little acts of kindness that make illness bearable, and be thankful for them.

- *Give back* to the NHS and your carers by providing thanks and constructive feedback. Share vital information with other patients and carers. Get involved in research, service improvement and design and volunteering for your local NHS and charities.

- *Eat well, Relax, Sleep* – even more important when you're ill.

The CLANGERS model equally applies to staff engagement and wellbeing. Health systems will always be high pressure places to work and so need to comprise of resilient organisations that support the mental health of the staff, encourage learning, are free from fear, bullying and blame and encourage everyone – patients, carers and staff alike – to speak up, feedback and continuously improve.

Ultimately, patients and carers must be handed as much control and responsibility as they want, and supported to live lives governed by their own goals and values, not the mass-produced end points of clinical trials. The best population evidence has to be combined with empathy for the individual. There is no single structure for healthcare provision that works in any context, and to continually seek the perfect structure in the NHS has proven to be hugely disruptive and disastrous for morale. Different models and structures will work in different parts of the country, but they must be built around common values and understanding of the needs of the individual. If each person can go about their daily CLANGERS, united by compassion, candour, competence and collaboration, then we can rediscover a values based service that is also effective and affordable.

CLANGERS in action and service re-design

I currently work in an NHS service for children and adolescents with chronic fatigue syndrome. I see new patients and their families in 90-minute consultations which gives me time to connect with them, explore their symptoms, concerns and lives in depth, make a diagnosis, be honest about the uncertainties that surround the illness, find out what matters most to them, acknowledge the difficulties they face, help them understand and interpret their condition in the context of their life circumstances, motivate them to want to change aspects of their lives that might be harming them, negotiate and agree a plan of action, and hand over as much information and responsibility self-care as they are willing and able to accept. I find my job incredibly rewarding and the feedback we receive is very positive. The thought of returning to 10-minute consultations as a GP fills me with dread.

Most of our service is provided by a team of occupational therapists, physiotherapists and psychologists, and we are aiming to collaborate across the NHS to serve children in areas that are currently poorly served. The following is the future vision of our service, and potentially other services, written by my consultant, Dr Esther Crawley.

Paediatric chronic fatigue syndrome (CFS/ME). This illness is relatively common (1-2.5% of children)[1] and potentially devastating.[2] Most children who access specialist services have been ill for over 18 months and attend less than two days of school.[3] About 50% of children are bed-bound at some stage[4] and therefore mothers often reduce or stop work with a negative impact on psychosocial well-being and family finances.[12] Whilst children and families access both secondary and tertiary health care, they experience barriers to diagnosis and treatment.[5]

Treatment for paediatric CFS/ME is highly effective. Between 66% and 85% of children will recover with specialist treatment at six months compared with 8% who do not get specialist treatment.[6] Whilst this should be good news for children with CFS/ME, few in the UK are able to access local specialist care. Children with CFS/ME are ill and their symptoms are frequently made worse by car travel so they are often unable to travel to distant specialist services. Sending out tertiary specialists to provide distant clinics is an expensive use of a limited resource and specialists do not have the local knowledge to develop an integrated care plan.

Our solution has been to recruit local therapists to be part of the specialist team delivering specialist treatment locally using a franchise model of care. Therapists receive training and supervision to obtain and maintain competences in the same way as all team members. Supervision is delivered using phone/Skype and occasional face to face contact. Therapists from satellite clinics attend team meetings either in person or using Skype. As with all franchise models, the satellite clinics collect outcome measures, use the same paperwork, leaflets and other tools as any other members of the team. They offer research opportunities to eligible patients as in the main centre enabling us to test interventions across a range of locations.

There are many advantages to this model of care. Patients benefit as they are able to access specialist knowledge locally. The specialist therapists are integrated within the local healthcare system and continue to work with the local provider. As they know the different agencies in the area, each child is more likely to obtain an integrated package of care. The families benefit as they do not need to travel and treatment means the child is more likely to return to school and the mother to work. Therapists benefit as they obtain specialist skills and are part of a nationally recognised service improving recruitment and retention. Patients and specialist therapists have almost immediate access to the latest research findings distributed at team meetings. The local health economy benefits as patients are taken out of expensive clinics with consultants and are treated more appropriately and cost-effectively by therapists. This model is now listed in the Dalton Review (page 23) as a model to consider in the future.

Developing this satellite model of delivering care to adolescents has forced us to find a variety of solutions to ensure quality is maintained, training delivered and the more complex cases are identified, triaged and signposted to the appropriate local or national provider.

Collection of routine patient-reported outcomes from the main hub and satellite clinics can support benchmarking and help quality control. This can now be done online using systems such as REDCap or equivalent NHS systems. We ask participants to complete patient-reported outcomes for us online and have used this successfully to benchmark services. Most systems have automated emails with individual secure links taking away a task from busy NHS clinicians. In the future we plan to link patient-reported outcome measures to online treatment (for example on line CBT) and the collection of harder data including exercise and hours of asleep. This could be adapted to other conditions and patients could download HR monitoring, BP monitoring, etc.

Skype and video conferencing can be used for training and supervision but also to provide assessments by other members of the team if patients are complex or specialist therapists want to access the multi-disciplinary team. Adolescents prefer Skype or video conferencing to telephone calls for consultations as it is more personal and meaningful. It seems likely that adults will feel the same way.

Paediatric CFS/ME is not the only long-term condition that suffers from a lack of local specialist care delivering effective and cost effective therapy. This type of model could be used for other long-term paediatric conditions including: child and adolescent mental healthcare, diabetes self-care, chronic pain services and obesity. In adults, this model could be used for CFS/ME, rheumatology services and chronic pain to name a few.

Conclusion: competent, compassionate, cost-effective collaboration

In the 31 years since I first set foot on an NHS ward, I've lived through a dozen major structural reforms, more ideological than evidence-based, seldom embedded long enough to prove their worth before being uprooted by the next political vanity project. So I'm loathe to suggest any structural miracle pill for universal healthcare. Continuous evidence-based improvement is far more likely to work, raising the quality bar a little at a time, as resources allow. Consultations – or rather meetings between experts – must be long enough to be safe, effective, enjoyable and meaningful. Transparency and accountability must embrace innovation and learning from failure. The spirit of competent and compassionate collaboration must triumph over competition.

Patients and carers must have as much choice and control over their illnesses as they – and a fair system – can manage. Anyone must feel free to speak up and challenge, knowing their concerns will be acted on. Pure knowledge, like pure water, must be available to all who need it. Communities must promote health and meaningful work for all, and we should all be taught the skills of resilience from a young age. The healthy must accept responsibility for trying to remain so, and society must support them. Artificial divisions must melt away (self-care, healthcare and social care are all care). And all of this care must be prudent, and mindful of the cost for the planet and the payer. The minimum necessary intervention is usually the kindest and the least obstructive. We have but one wild and precious life, and we want healthcare to improve us, not imprison us. Release the joy of your inner CLANGERS.

With thanks to Dr Esther Crawley

Renewing centre-left Labour Party politics and policy for the NHS and health

Paul Corrigan

This chapter is primarily about politics and only secondly about policy. Given the profoundly political nature of the NHS in England, politics and policy are always heavily intertwined. However most policy is written as if the good ideas that the policy contains can in some way be abstracted from the messy business of politics and implemented in their pure nature. It can't.

Despite many lamentations to the contrary the NHS is essentially political. It was born completely out of politics. Very many people thrill to an enormous political narrative that created the NHS. In 1948 a country bankrupt from the war and the fight against Nazism redefined itself around a health service that was paid for by everyone out of national taxation and aimed to provide equal access for all, irrespective of wealth. People love this deeply political story of its birth but then they lament the fact that the NHS is political.

Without politics there would be no NHS. It has been developed, maintained and revived through political activity. The national taxation that keeps it going is raised every year through the votes of national politicians deciding to spend the public's money on the NHS and not elsewhere. And, if any right-wing political party ever manages it, then the NHS would also be killed off because of politics.

This is not just a chapter about politics but a particular strain of politics within the Labour Party. Variously called the centre left, social democrat and for a brief historical spell New Labour. From within that tradition I work through the main themes of what a centre-left politics of the NHS will mean in the near future.

For most of those involved in democratic politics September 2015 (the month of the deadline for this chapter) has been an important month. The election of Jeremy Corbyn as leader of the Labour Party and the resulting advocacy of an open and deep debate about politics and policy has radically changed my approach to these ideas. Over the last 10 years I and my colleagues on the centre left have failed to publicly engage in this debate because of anxieties about unity of purpose. This was a self-induced mistake.

In these last few weeks we are being encouraged to think wider and deeper than we have done for a very long time and I want to try to live up to that injunction in this chapter. I engage in this debate from a particular history in the politics and policy of the NHS and health in England. Between 2001 and 2007 I was a special adviser to Alan Milburn, John Reid and Tony Blair – all strong advocates of New Labour. I worked with them and was very happy to develop New Labour policy and politics.

What we were doing then was renewing Labour's long-term approach to the NHS and health. We are now eight years on from the end of that period. What I learnt from that political period is not that the politics and policy from that time and place would be the ones that would guide us for the next 50 years. What I learnt from then is that it is vital to be in a position to revise politics and policy in the light of new problems and issues. As this chapter will show, the principles you apply can be constant but the problems you apply them to will be very different.

Therefore, in September 2015 we will not go back to 2008 and read forward what we did then into now. What was 'new' then is pretty old now. So here I want to start that renewing process over again in a very new set of circumstances.

There are five issues I want to develop:

1. Equality of access is an important principle for the NHS but it's much more important as a practice. To develop better equality of access for the public the NHS needs to reform.

2. A better NHS with more equal access needs more active citizens, a more active public and more active patients.

3. The NHS on its own cannot improve healthcare, it needs partners; new forms of provision will need new organisers of that provision.

4. However big the NHS is it can only improve health in partnership with others. Men and women make their own health but not under conditions of their own choosing.

5. Since taxation will be the only way of raising money for the NHS, waste and inefficiency increase patient distress and risk lives.

1. Equality of access is an important principle for the NHS but it's much more important as a practice. To develop better equality of access for the public the NHS needs to reform.

As in 2000, the first and most important political issue is how we approach in 2015 the basic principles of the NHS. In 2000 the NHS Plan was clear. The 2000 NHS Plan starts from the idea that providing equal access for all, free at the point of need and paid for out of national taxation, was so important that we needed to deliver it in practice.

Everyone across the political spectrum 'believes' in the principles behind the NHS. From Nigel Farage to Jeremy Corbyn, that belief unites politicians. What was different in the NHS Plan was a recognition that the principle was not being met. Waiting over a year for a heart operation was not what the principle of the NHS was all about. The NHS Plan recognised if we wanted to make that principle a reality then the NHS as a set of delivery mechanisms would have to radically change.

Over the years many people on the left confuse the aspiration of equal access for all with the reality of that equal access being met. They believe that once the NHS removed the necessity of reaching into your post office book to buy healthcare, this provided equal access. It didn't and it hasn't. Removing the privilege of money in access has been vital, but it has not on its own provided equal access for all.

For decades, despite healthcare being free at the point of need, Tudor Hart's inverse care law that poorer people need more healthcare and yet get poorer healthcare has run through the NHS. Between 2000 and 2010 the very boring issue of decreasing the maximum waiting times for diagnosis and treatment increased the equality of access to NHS care. It could only be achieved by getting the NHS to take seriously the public demand to have quicker access to healthcare. And achieving that took a lot of reform of NHS delivery services.

Many people on the left disagreed with the process of reforming the NHS. Whilst the left sees itself as radical on so many issues, on the NHS it is essentially conservative. New Labour in 2000 was radical because it wanted the NHS to apply those egalitarian principles in practice and not just in theory.

This strange conservatism is still there from the left in 2015. My only explanation for this is that the left fears that the NHS – as a set of funding and delivery principles which are separate from most other politics and policies in England – is in some way fragile. And because of this fragility, we all need to step around the organisation quietly, thanking it for doing so well and not being open to criticism and reform.

My take on this is very different. I am the same age as the NHS and through my life I have seen it grow and develop as a major part of British society. One of the main successes of New Labour is that after 13 years in power, by 2010 a larger proportion of the electorate agreed with its principles than ever before. This is a very powerful institution which needs and demands critical friends rather than fawning adulation.

In 2015 providing equal access for all for the 17 million people with long-term conditions will require very radical change to the way in which the NHS and social care delivery mechanism have been set up. The NHS like has been set up to deal with a different demographics and different diseases. Holding the NHS still will not achieve this.

One of the main political differences within the left is a belief among some that it is the role of the state and its organisations alone to ensure greater equality. The post-war welfare state created very large state institutions to abolish Beveridge's five devils of idleness, squalor, ignorance, want and disease. Each of these very large post-war institutions – full employment, state housing, secondary education for all, social security and the NHS made very great strides in reducing inequalities. But on their own they did not succeed in creating equal access or equality of opportunity, let alone equality of outcomes. Indeed the history of post-1960 English politics is a history of rediscovering inequalities in income, housing, education and health. For the left this rediscovery demands greater and greater state effort.

For the centre left greater equality demands the greater activity of families and communities in working with the state to tackle these issues. The state cannot take all the agency; people need to take that agency.

From the 1950s it was true that hundreds of thousands of council houses helped to raise families above the squalor of the 1930s. But without the hard work of families turning these houses into homes, the limitations of what the state could achieve by constructing buildings became obvious in the next couple of decades.

Full employment created the conditions where greater wealth could be earned in wages and salaries, but it was the hard work of women and men in those jobs working evenings and weekends that gained the extra resources to build a better life.

Secondary education for all – more and better teachers and schools – created the conditions for better educational opportunities, but without the aspiration and hard work of pupils, parents and their communities in learning, very little happens in these buildings.

And the same is true in health and the health service. Active patients make better healthcare. Agency must not be taken from people by state services. Passive patients will not have the agency to improve their own conditions or their own health.

Here we need to rethink the problem that appears to be posed by the NHS of 'rising expectations' as a problem. Every other industry sees rising expectations as a resource and not a problem. For the NHS to thrive it needs to welcome this increased expectation and try to universalise it.

2. A better NHS with more equal access needs more active citizens, a more active public, and more active patients.

For at least the last 20 years the politicians responsible for the NHS have argued that the NHS needs to be more patient-centred. In a lot of change this has been consistent. Whilst there has been a bit of a shift, by and large very few patients and indeed no politician would say that all of this political endeavour has borne fruit. By and large power in the NHS, either for citizens or patients, is very similar to where it was two decades ago.

Given this record of failure (and let's be clear my own period of working in Whitehall had no better record of concrete patient empowerment than any other), why do I think the next few years will be any different? And why do I believe that centre-left politics will play an important role in these developments?

The argument for a patient-empowered NHS has been mainly ideological. Given the importance of health in everyone's lives, then greater control of health and healthcare would be a good thing in itself. But this moral argument for change appears to have bounced off the NHS as a healthcare system and made very little impact.

What is different now and for the future is that this ideological argument for change has been joined by a material need for change. The NHS, as with nearly every other healthcare system in the world, is facing a very changed pattern of disease. The 17 million people in England with long-term conditions, who use about two-thirds of the resources of the NHS, now have the main burden of disease. Over the next decade they will be joined by millions of others with multiple long-term conditions, some of whom are the first generation in their families to live beyond 85 and will have two or three of these long-term conditions.

The success of acute care services in the NHS has changed the outcomes of what were the great killers of the previous 50 years. In the 1950s, if an uncle had a heart attack he died. Sixty years on nearly everyone survives their first heart attack and then lives on with heart trouble. Halfway through 2006 the majority of people who had cancer started to survive beyond five years.

The fact that killing diseases have now become something that most survive is a wonderful advance for individuals and for people as a whole. Let's be clear that for the British public there is no downside to this.

The outcome is that what have been killing diseases become long-term conditions for what we hope are the rest of patient's long lives. In demand for healthcare terms these successes are adding to that demand every day. As we improve stroke care and other diseases we will continue to add the demand for long-term care for those older people that survive.

How does this change the politics of a patient-centred NHS? First, this increased demand for healthcare is not a future statistic. It is happening now in the increased demand for GP appointments and with the increased demand for in-patient emergency care beds for older, sicker people.

Second, the secret to the radical solution is in the phrase long-term. Those of us with these conditions have them for a long time, usually for life. That means that patients experience the condition over a long time. If I have arthritis or breathing problems, for example, I have the opportunity to really come to know a lot about my condition, and how it interacts with my body, mind and life. If I am quite ill with my long-term condition, I might see the NHS for 20 hours every year when they are 'in charge' of my health but, for the other 5,800-plus waking hours a year, I am in charge together with my family and friends.

The secret for the future of the NHS is that the NHS either recognises that I am in charge for nearly all of the time and invests in my capacity to manage my long-term condition, or it denies this, claiming to be in charge of my health throughout the year and tries to run it from those 20 hours.

These material facts make the argument for giving patients more power over their healthcare. If the NHS can manage the profound change contained in this it will survive and even thrive. If it does not, the NHS will increasingly buckle as it tries to take all the responsibility for the greater and greater ill health in our society.

This might appear a no-brainer. But actually the NHS finds this transformation very hard. It is profoundly ambivalent about how it should interact with the increased burden of ill health. On the one hand it argues that patients should look after themselves more and the NHS will spend some time in a consultation telling people they should exercise more, eat differently and drink less. It will then despair that when they next see the patient they have not done as they are told. If only patients did as they were told they would not need to come and see me as often. Instinctively the NHS knows that patients have power over their demand for healthcare.

But on the other hand, the NHS sees the primary care system in this country not as one that is dominated and run by patients, their families and their communities, but one that is run by the NHS. If primary (initial, prime, crucial: all synonyms for the word primary) care meant anything, it would be the care system that the patient works with in their lives over those 5,800-plus waking hours when they are managing their own diseases. The job of the NHS would be to invest in the capacity of people and their carers and communities, to better manage their condition. This would involve the use of modern technology and patient and community education and links with the strong network of community organisations and patient groups that exist. It does not come free. It would cost some money.

Given the immense strain upon the existing GP services as the current primary care system, you would think that the NHS would welcome this. However, their response to this increased burden of disease is to make the case out for more of the same resource. If current demand is met with seven-minute slots of GP time, then we work out how many extra slots we will need for the extra demand and, bingo, that gives us the number of extra GPs we simply must have to continue the service as it is.

The idea of taking some of the money that is spent on what is seen as the current primary care system and investing it in the real primary care system runs into the limits of radicalism within the structures of the NHS.

And this is where politics comes in. Even given the obvious material case for increased investment in the patient's capacity to better manage their long-term condition, left to itself the NHS will not make this paradigm shift in what counts as care. The adulation of the existing delivery system I mentioned above will not bring about a patient-centred system.

One of the ways that this will happen irretrievably would be to greatly increase the range and number of those patients who have an individual health budget. Over the last couple of decades over 600,000 people in social care have been given their local authority budget to run their own care services. In 2015 some small examples of personal health budgets were being piloted. Giving people control of the NHS money that would be spent on their long-term condition, and through that money the support services that they buy for themselves, would radically change the balance of power in favour of the patient.

Given the importance of empowerment to centre-left politics, the very rapid extension of these pilots to the millions of people who experience long-term conditions would mark the reform that is most likely to empower patients to better manage their long-term conditions. Given the dislocation that will be experienced by the NHS if millions of patients were buying their own care and support, left to itself the NHS will not do this. It will be the politics of empowerment that will drive the policies that create that empowerment.

3. The NHS on its own cannot improve healthcare, it needs partners; new forms of provision will need new organisers of that provision.

Given the NHS is the biggest institution in England, it thinks it makes the weather and needs little help from others. Compared with local government it has a poor history of making partnerships with others. Yet the tasks now facing it demand much better and broader partnerships.

Apart from empowering patients, their carers and communities to add more value to their own healthcare, the NHS and other services also need to change the way in which they organise provision for people with long-term conditions.

Existing provision is organised around the healthcare specialists that have developed within the NHS over the last 70 years. The NHS, for the best of reasons, has fragmented care between primary care, tens of different specialisms within secondary acute physical care, mental healthcare and community care. Each of these institutions have deep expertise in their specialism that can impact upon specific disease patterns.

The new disease burden however lies with those patients with long-term conditions who develop more than one condition. Specialist care leaves the 85-year-old with breathing problems, diabetes and depression trying to organise several different specialists, often working from several different institutions. Each of these specialists may be world class, but no-one is treating the whole patient and putting that patient at the centre of their own care.

This leads to duplication and confusion which is why the NHS has been given such a strong push towards the need for person-centred integrated care. Organising these specialists to work together in the interest of the patient is proving a task that appears beyond most of the existing NHS institutions. Over the last few years, despite many attempts at innovation, the vast majority of NHS and social care practice remains stubbornly fragmented.

The much wider spread of individual health budgets to millions of people with long-term conditions would have an impact on this. Buying their own care with NHS money would potentially put the patient in command of their care. It would, however, be a difficult task for patients on their own to integrate the very high status doctors who provide specialist care from specialist hospitals into a patient pathway organised around the patient's life. Getting patient care organised around the patient and not the existing NHS organisation will take a shift in power.

For this, active patients will need new organisations that will take the lead in coordinating what are, at present, fragmented NHS institutions and working beyond the NHS with social care and other support from the voluntary sector.

Existing patient organisations have the trust and the capacity to step up to this task. Organisations such as Macmillan for cancer care and the British Heart Foundation for heart disease already provide services for NHS patients. They know the problems with the existing fragmentation of NHS care and have a deep knowledge of the day-to-day needs of their patients for coordinated care.

The development of person-centred coordinated care will need them to take on the task of better coordinating care amongst all these institutions currently providing fragmented care. They have the trust of patients; they have the trust of many clinicians and they could develop the capacity to organise existing fragmented services into person-centred pathways. As voluntary organisations themselves they would work well with those parts of the voluntary sector that would help better management of care. Organisationally they would act as accountable lead providers to contracts that have been commissioned to provide coordinated care for people with long-term conditions.

They would work directly, with the patients who have individual budgets, to provide care that was coordinated around their needs and not the needs of existing organisations.

4. However big the NHS is, it can only improve health in partnership with others. Men and women make their own health but not under conditions of their own choosing.

The politics of public health that swings between a non-interventionist right wing and an interventionist left wing has consistently missed the point about our lives and our health. For too long the public health service has been confused with the public's health. Whilst the former is an important aspect of our services, it is the latter that really matters. If we are to empower the public in playing a bigger role in their own health service then we must start off by recognising that they own their own health.

Of course, people make their own health under different conditions and we need to work with them to change those conditions. The day-by-day struggle of individuals and families to improve their life conditions is an important part of gaining more control over their lives. People will only be in charge of their own health if they are in charge of other aspects of their lives.

Over generations, working with people individually and collectively to change the economic and social conditions that restrict them has been one of the guiding aims of the centre left. As I outlined above, many millions of people have worked hard with educational and economic opportunities to change the conditions under which they and their families live their lives. This has not been done for people by the state but through a joint set of activities between the hard work of people and the opportunity provided by the public services.

The same will happen with health improvement. We need to more clearly understand the very specific motivations around health improvement that are contained in the different groups and communities in our society. People will engage in improving their own and their community's health when they see the point. Not when we tell them to.

5. Since taxation will be the only way of raising money for the NHS, waste and inefficiency increase patient distress and risks lives.

Politics will mean that in the near future there will be no new co-payments to bolster the NHS resources that come from taxation. We need to recognise that economic growth will be the only way of increasing NHS funding. It's true that in 2002 it was possible to increase national insurance contributions to pay for an increase in NHS resources. But most of the doubling of resources for the NHS that took place between 1997 and 2010 came from the proceeds of economic growth.

After the international financial crash in 2008 the economics of our country will be different from the 10 years before that international crisis. It is therefore difficult to see the economy growing in the next 10 years to the same extent it did after 1997. This means that for the next 10 years at least, the NHS is going to be very short of money. Demand – especially from long-term conditions – will increase faster than the finances that come from taxation.

This is a problem for serious centre-left political parties across the world. We no longer have the opportunity to increase public expenditure on the back of fast economic growth. That means for serious political parties we need a different relationship to public spending. It still remains, as it always was, an important method of developing services to increase equality of opportunity that would otherwise be blocked by purely private distribution. It is now, however, a much more scarce resource to be valued, pound for pound, much more highly than in a time of plenty.

This will need a moral shift in the way the NHS spends the public's money. We need to make sure that for everyone in the NHS – staff and patients – any waste or inefficiency is seen as an attack upon the basic principle of the NHS. In a time of scarcity wasting a few million pounds will lead to reduction in the equal access for all and an increase in distress amongst the sick.

Whilst currently efficiency and the elimination of waste is seen as a management task – given that whenever any waste occurs for any reason it will lead to harm for a potential patient in not saving that resource – it now becomes everyone's business.

Waste is there in its billions because of inefficient procurement. Waste is also there in its billions because of what health services call allocative inefficiency. This is where patients are inappropriately being treated by an expensive healthcare provider when they should be better treated by a cheaper one.

The most significant of this is where many thousands of nights in hospitals are spent in emergency in-patient beds – emergencies that happen because (as outlined above) too many older people have had insufficient investment in their capacity to better manage their own conditions at home. Very, very few of these patients want to leave their own bed for a hospital bed but at the moment the allocative inefficiency of the NHS means they end up in the most expensive and least wanted place.

Conclusion

For the last few years the centre-left has given over the politics of the NHS to the conservative left. This has been our fault. After years of practical improvement on issues such as waiting times, we have become much too technocratic in the policies we have advocated.

The passion for improving the capacity of the NHS to work with people to improve their lives does not come from a conservative left that sees the state as the answer to everything. In the past we have recognised the importance of personal and collective agency in improving the lives of our citizens. The centre-left will now refind its political passion for helping to develop more active patients with the NHS and social care services.

Unsurprisingly this will need radical change to the way in which the NHS works. That change will need the new policies that I have outlined above. However, over the next few years the development of a coherent and passionate centre-left politics for the NHS will be vital for both the NHS and for politics. In a few years' time we will look back on this recent period of political silence by the centre-left as a brief aberration for these politics.

Commissioning the future

Stephen Dorrell

The NHS provides examples of the best aspects of the British approach to life, and the worst.

To start with the positives, the NHS is an expression of values which are embraced across our society. The principle that access to care should be available, means blind, to those who need it receives virtually unanimous support in Britain, because it is seen – rightly in my view – to represent the application of the principles of social justice to the world of healthcare. Equitable access to high quality care, based on individual need and clinical priority, are at the very heart of our sense of justice and fairness, and we are offended when individuals who need care find themselves unable to access it.

Furthermore, the NHS is not just an expression of values; the organisations which make up the NHS deliver care which is near the top of most international comparisons of quality and efficiency. The NHS is not, as it is sometimes portrayed, a pampered and inefficient elite, insulated from real life; in fact most of the people it employs are motivated by a desire to deliver good quality and efficient care and they take seriously both their professional duty to patients and their stewardship duty to taxpayers.

And yet, while recognising its undoubted successes, the NHS can also illustrate some of our less attractive national characteristics.

Unsurprisingly, given our geography, we are prone to be insular. In some moods this leads us to celebrate the fact that our geography has given us the self-confidence to develop a global view; we see ourselves as natural individualists with innovation in our blood. But in our less attractive moments we allow our insularity to convince us that our circumstances are unique and that differences between our approach and other people's simply need to be explained rather than questioned.

It is, therefore, one thing to recognise that the NHS is a success story in international terms; it is quite another to be so convinced by the narrative of NHS success that our minds resist new ideas on the grounds, spoken or unspoken, that they weren't invented here. No healthcare system is perfect, but we can learn something from most of them – which is why I believe it is so important that the NHS is not allowed simply to explain to itself why it is different.

Both good stewardship and our duty to patients require us to be constantly challenged to learn from experience – which means both our own experience which is often not applied consistently, and the experience of other countries who face similar health and social issues.

It is this requirement for constant and effective challenge which lies at the heart of the function of commissioners. It is of course a familiar argument – first heard in the NHS in the late 1980s when Ken Clarke proposed the introduction of what was then described as 'the purchaser/provider split'. It was hugely controversial at the time and remained so when, bizarrely, both the Blair government (in 2002) and the Coalition government (in 2012) felt the urge to re-legislate the same idea, claiming on each occasion that it was a decisive break with the past. In 1990 it was truly new; thereafter the surrounding political noise obscured the underlying truth that the purchaser/provider principle, now known as commissioner/provider has been settled government policy for over a quarter of a century.

For a principle which has been at the heart of public policy for so long it is surprising how poorly it is understood – and how little serious thought has, until recently, been devoted to it.

It is, for example, often confused with the related but different argument about delegated management of providers. This argument, encapsulated in the principle of foundation trusts, stresses the importance of empowered delegated management structures. Although it has also been subject to attack from opponents who have asserted that it represents 'backdoor privatisation' and causes 'fragmentation' or 'marketisation' of service, neither proposition is true. The argument for delegated and empowered management is little more than the application of the principles of good management to healthcare organisations.

There is extensive evidence which demonstrates that organisations achieve better staff motivation and more efficient use of resources when they empower local management. Delegated structures are designed simply to introduce these basic management ideas into the delivery of NHS services – and it is striking that the opposition to this principle has now largely evaporated.

The same cannot be said of the role of commissioners. This question is both difficult and important because it focuses on the question that the advocates of delegated management do not address. Even if it is accepted that delegated structures produce better management, this acceptance does not address the questions of purpose and accountability. Who determines the priorities and how is management held to account? How can locally managed organisations be knitted together into systems which deliver joined up care to those who rely on them in ways which respond to their changing needs and wishes.

The easy answer is that it is the role of commissioners, but few would argue that it has been successfully discharged. Indeed it is often argued that 'there is no evidence that commissioning adds value and it is time to recognize that it has failed'. The problem with this argument is that its proponents have nothing to put in its place.

Some argue that what is required is a return to a hierarchical national structure which determines priorities and coordinates local organisations. We should be careful what we wish for. Instead of longing for a mythical status quo ante, where flexible organisations responded to far sighted leadership, I prefer to remember how we got here and ask why commissioning has not been as effective as we hoped.

The first and most obvious answer to that question is that commissioning has been the subject of obsessional organisational churn. The process of repeated re-legislation of the idea through reshaped institutions has been very destructive of the understanding and goodwill on which effective commissioning depends. Each new manifestation has required management to recreate teams which have been charged with applying a marginally different version of the same idea in a different geography. It has meant that commissioners have had no choice but to spend time building and rebuilding processes rather than using and developing these processes to improve care. It has been a classic case of 'pulling up the plant to see if the roots are growing'.

This persistent immaturity of commissioning processes has also had secondary effects which have compounded the problem.

Institutional churn has led many experienced NHS managers to take opportunities for early retirement or career change which has resulted in a well-documented shortage of experienced senior managers. This has been a problem across the NHS, but it has been particularly acutely felt in commissioning structures which have often appeared to offer more precarious and less fulfilling roles.

This immaturity has also led commissioners to retreat into a massively legalistic and bureaucratised version of competition in healthcare services. The arguments about competition have been presented in a highly politicised environment in terms which suggest that competition and collaboration are alternatives and there is a choice to be made.

I do not believe that either proposition is true. Human beings are naturally competitive, and the urge to find new and better ways to treat patients and organise services is a fact of life and a force for good. The question is how to harness that natural energy in ways which recognise the undoubted need for collaboration between different individuals, teams and organisations if we are to deliver the core objective of equitable access to high quality services.

The most fundamental weakness of current structures is that they encourage us to treat care as a series of unrelated transactions, dealing with specific conditions, and they undervalue the connections both between the experiences of service users and within services providers. This tendency to fragment services into apparently unrelated transactions has the effect of undermining both quality and efficiency in the delivery of service.

As a long-term supporter of the argument for commissioning it is important not to deny the force of these arguments. They reflect the experience of many who have operated the system for over 25 years as well as the observable fact that our care system is not joined up in the way that it should be. Simply to deny that the commissioning process has any responsibility for these facts is to rely on assertion rather than evidence.

The right response is to recognise there is truth in the argument and ask whether it invalidates the commissioning approach, or whether the performance of commissioners can be improved by changing practice. I strongly believe the second is the right approach. The challenge is to develop an approach to commissioning which preserves the principle of effective challenge to present and future service providers while responding to the requirement for a more collaborative approach to service delivery.

Recent history demonstrates why these issues are best addressed by evolutionary change. As we have seen, commissioning has remained stunted within the NHS, in part because of protracted periods of institutional uncertainty, and the commitment to evolutionary development which lies at the heart of the Five Year Forward View provides a clear and welcome opportunity for a new and more sophisticated approach to commissioning to emerge.

The opportunity should be seized with both hands, but what are the essential characteristics of success?

Firstly, after over 70 years of rhetoric, it is high time that we shifted our priorities to focus less on rationing access to treatment and more on enabling citizens to lead healthy and enjoyable lives. Public health should not be an afterthought; it should be at the heart of policymaking.

This is why, although there are some adjustment pains, I believe the transfer of public health responsibility under the 2012 Act to Public Health England and local government was an important improvement in the structure of public policy. Public Health England has still to learn and apply the lesson that no minister has the power to silence well-evidenced public health interventions; it needs to develop the institutional self-confidence to speak truth unto power and call national government to account for the health impact of its decisions across the range of its activities.

Directors of public health (DPH) should perform the same role within local government. Public health is not a discrete service line; it is a way of thinking about public policy – it should engage with planning, housing, education and employment issues as well as focusing on outcomes achieved by the local health and care sector. The DPH should be part of local decision making, and yet apart from it; willing to participate in shaping decisions while preserving the freedom to call those decisions to account in the forum of public opinion.

When the director of public health is performing this role effectively, there will be a close link with the work of the commissioner of health and care services. It is the DPH who will identify priorities, compare outcomes and challenge the commissioner. Why are outcomes for condition X in Newcastle worse than in Bristol or Hamburg? Why is the incidence of condition Y greater in Norwich than in Lichfield or Charleston? An effective DPH will provide a running commentary on the performance of the commissioner, and will ensure that if they are minded to live with a sub-optimal solution they will need to prepare themselves to explain it to a sceptical DPH.

Second, commissioners of future services need to prepare themselves for a fundamentally different relationship with citizens. This is partly the result of the rising expectation that tax-funded services should treat them with the same respect that they experience and expect in the rest of their lives, and it is partly the realisation that 'health' is not something dispensed by clinicians, but the result of multiple decisions, many of which impact directly on an individual's quality of life as well as creating the context in which they experience a need for care. Commissioners need to learn to work with citizens to support the lives they want to lead, rather than trying to substitute their choices for those made by citizens.

A third challenge for commissioners is to break down the traditional silos within which public services work. To take a simple example, how can it possibly make sense to think about pediatric services, without engaging with schools and children's social services? How is it possible to plan the future of social services without engaging with social housing providers, as well as the NHS? Similarly, is it possible to develop effective drug and alcohol services without engaging with the police and criminal justice system?

Commissioners of the future must therefore look beyond traditional silos. Just as public health has become part of the fabric of local government, so the different commissioning processes which shape local public health services, including the NHS, must become embedded in the functions of local government. Local authorities are not primarily service providers; they are the means by which local people make decisions about the shape of their communities in the future. They should be, to use the fashionable word, the catalyst which encourages valuable local collaboration.

If local authorities develop this role they will find there are two further groups of stakeholders whose opinions will need to be reflected in their decisions about the future shape of health and care services.

The first of these is the professional community. In recent years it has been fashionable to emphasise the role of GPs, on the grounds that within the NHS it is often (but not always) the GP who is best placed to see the service from the patient's point of view. But if the commissioner of future services is to reshape services to respond to the priorities of those who use them, it is important that they are able to call on the full range of relevant professional expertise; they should use the commissioning process to introduce external professional expertise, for example in hospital medicine and social work, to examine local outcomes and challenge local practitioners to improve them.

The second key group is voters. The defining characteristic of services provided for a commissioner is that they are paid for, at least in part, by taxpayers. Whether seen primarily as taxpayers, and therefore paymasters, or simply as voters in local democracy, commissioners of health and care services should expect to give account of themselves to the local community. Embedding these decisions within the functions of local government will be an important step in creating a more healthy balance between national and local accountability for health and care services.

It is this requirement to improve the accountability of public services to local communities which represents the most powerful agent of change in Britain today – and is the reason why it is important to develop a more coherent view of the role of the commissioner in the development of modern public services.

We know the NHS needs to develop a more collaborative service model but the real challenge is to follow through the logic of that commitment; we shall not build more collaborative services by allowing the NHS to retreat into its comfort zone. The key to success lies in local commissioners, looking across the range of public services, and challenging the health and care sector (of which the NHS is an important part, but not the whole) to deliver collaboration, not just with itself but with the full range of local public services.

That is why current developments in Manchester are so important. I do not argue that Manchester will get everything right (it won't), or that the Manchester model will work everywhere (that isn't true either). What is true however is that the logic of Manchester is universal.

At the heart of the Manchester approach is the belief that commissioners of public services in a place have more in common with each other than any has with any service provider. In other words the relationship between NHS commissioners and social housing commissioners spending 'Manchester pounds' to deliver 'Manchester public services' is more important than the relationship between the NHS commissioner and a hospital or the social housing commissioner and a housing association. Each relationship is of course important, but it is the total impact of outcomes achieved for the citizens of Manchester which matters, rather than the history or interests of individual institutions.

It is a developing revolution in public services, and it holds out the hope of creating a new relationship between the citizen and the community in which they live – as well as a new relationship between commissioners and providers of services. That is why I have described Sir Howard Bernstein, the principle architect of 'Devo-Manc' as 'the new Beveridge'. It is important to UK citizens well beyond Manchester that his ideas prove to be as successful and as enduring as those which we still honour but which were first advanced over 80 years ago.

Three challenges for the future: funding, integration and the workforce

Richard Murray

The NHS remains one of England's most popular institutions and its staff amongst the most respected professions in the country.[1] The extent of support for the NHS becomes even more remarkable when we look overseas: the Commonwealth Fund surveys of international healthcare systems continue to underline the exceptional regard of the British for the NHS.[2] Lastly – and perhaps even more surprising to commentators – the NHS in 2015 is also seen by many of the public to be performing well against its own historical track record.[3]

When thinking about the future for the NHS, this might lead us to conclude 'if it ain't broke, don't fix it'. There is certainly an element of truth in this given the public in general do not see anything fundamentally wrong with the NHS and, as such, reformers should avoid tampering with its fundamental principles.

However, preserving the founding principles of the NHS – a (largely) free at the point of use, tax-funded, comprehensive service – is not the same as rejecting all change. The NHS and its sister service, social care, both face some old challenges and some new ones. Many of these are well rehearsed: an ageing population with increasing numbers of long-term conditions, patchy integration with social care, and persistent health inequalities linked with a stubborn set of public health problems such as obesity that threaten the future health of the population. Many of these challenges underpin the recent Five Year Forward View launched by the array of NHS national bodies and the reform programme we are currently experiencing.[4]

Rather than rehearse the Five Year Forward View I will set out instead three key areas where making further progress would help deliver the change we need and preserve those founding principles of the NHS that the British public continues to value so strongly. These three areas are funding, integration and the workforce.

Funding

In all developed nations, healthcare is expensive and it eats up a substantial and usually growing share of national income.[5] This international perspective is important: without it, we could wrongly come to the conclusion that the NHS is expensive. It is not – compared to many of our international partners whether, for example, this is the US, Canada, Germany or France – the UK spends relatively little on healthcare. Not only that, but if the government's spending plans are realised we will spend less in 2020 than we did in 2005 as a share of GDP creating an unprecedented decade-long slowdown in health spending.[6]

Given the stresses and strains we can already see in the NHS today, particularly in the rapid spread of deficits in NHS hospitals,[7] it may be that this spending restraint will prove impossible to maintain. Even so, the restraint we have already witnessed over 2010-2015 is remarkable and the promises of extra money for the NHS in the recent general election were all small by historic standards.

This points to one of the weaknesses of the UK tax-funded NHS. As part of wider public expenditure the NHS experiences (though admittedly less so than other parts of the public sector) the same booms and busts that buffet our public finances. Further, with the tax funding for the NHS simply part of the overall tax take, there is no easy way for the public to understand where their money goes. Adding spice to this mix, the political importance attached to the NHS makes its funding the subject of party politics which arguably does not help long-term planning and makes it difficult for the public to engage in, or even understand, the options they may have on funding for the NHS.

In a service like healthcare where it takes many years to alter health behaviours or train a new workforce, the lack of any future funding envelope can turn planning into guesswork. It can also make long-term investments like the workforce and public health vulnerable to short-term funding pressures. More generally, the stop-start track record of NHS finances in no way matches the changes in the nation's long-term demographics that determines the need for healthcare services and as we know, is steadily pushing up that demand over time.

It does not need to be this way. To provide both greater transparency and independence, the Bank of England was given power over monetary policy. To build credibility and independence the Office of Budget Responsibility (OBR) was given (a different) set of responsibilities over the forecasting of public finances. The NHS should have its own OBR to estimate the money it needs to provide a comprehensive set of services, free of boom and bust, and the government should commit to providing that money or explaining to the public why not. As well as providing greater stability and certainty over financing it would provide the public with a source of non-political information on the funding needs of the NHS. In the long-term it is unlikely that an OBR for health would by itself actually raise the level of spending (governments usually find themselves forced to provide the NHS with money when crises hit anyway), but if it does, at least it should be after a clear public debate. If there is any additional bill to be paid by the public sector, it is likely to come from social care but I will cover this when discussing integration.

Integration

The case for better integration between health and social care is both well made and well understood and needs no rehearsing here. Making real progress has, however, been harder to deliver. At least some of the reasons for this difficulty no doubt reflect the long-term separation between the two services and practical challenges of bringing two systems and cultures together at ground level. Many of the models being explored through the Five Year Forward View and other initiatives should be able to set out proven pathways to closer integration and, of course, the new devolution agenda pioneered in Greater Manchester also has integration as a core objective.[8]

However, this is unlikely to be enough. Local government has suffered the most from the need to balance the budget and the provision of social care in England has shrunk in consequence. It is difficult to integrate two services when one of them is facing significant, year-on-year cuts to its budgets. Attempts to use the NHS to provide financial support to social care, notably through the Better Care Fund, only work as long as the NHS has money to spare and this is no longer the case. Even without the reductions in social care, the fundamentally different financing philosophies underpinning the two systems will always make true integration hard.

In addition to progress on the best models to integrate care through the Five Year Forward View and other initiatives, the independent Barker Commission recommended that health and social care be brought together in a single ring-fenced budget and that over time, the gulf between the means-tested social care system and the free-at-the-point of use NHS be reduced by levelling up social care.[9]

This is right: the future NHS needs a well-functioning social care system and that cannot happen without providing both the money social care needs and by removing the existing funding barriers between the two systems in so far as this is possible. In the future we need to recognise that `healthcare' also needs to routinely encompass social care.

However, we also need a further dose of integration. At the moment, the usual response to the many persistent lifestyle issues we face as a nation – whether obesity, lack of physical activity, alcohol overuse or tobacco – is to look to the NHS to provide more advice and support on healthy lifestyles. There is of course no doubt an important role for these public health services, even if the 2012 reforms actually moved some of them over to local government and outside the formal definition of the `NHS'. Even classifying these devolved public health budgets as part of wider health spending still leaves many opportunities untapped in the wider public health agenda:

- The contribution the voluntary and community sector (VCS) can make to health and wellbeing has been recognised in some areas, but too often they remain on the boundaries of formal services and many barriers remain to proper joint working. It is one of the great opportunities for the future that the NHS, social care and the VCS will find a way to unlock proper co-production and this is true for health and healthcare;

- Health is not the preserve of healthcare services, not in England or indeed anywhere. Wider determinants of health often dominate the impact of formal health services and many (but not all) of these in England are the responsibility of local government.[10] Recognising and capitalising on these responsibilities and the benefit they can bring to health and wellbeing is one of the great opportunities for devolution, whether it be in housing, green spaces or environmental services;[11] and

- Lastly, better integration with the VCS and with other public services is primarily a local agenda. However, there are also important levers at national level, including regulation and tax. At least on anti-smoking policy the importance of regulation is well known and remains a potent tool to reduce the use of tobacco. However, elsewhere it is much less easy to see if the potential that regulation and tax policy could make to influencing people's choices is routinely considered. Whether in a possible tax on saturated fats, or regulations that can control access to alcohol, national policy making needs to show it has considered health in a more fundamental way and this could be a role for an enhanced Public Health England.

The benefits of integration in this wider sense is primarily about making the most of the assets and tools we already have. This should improve health and wellbeing. In some cases it may also make services cheaper – either by delivering them in a more efficient way or because, over time, it helps reduce the future demand for services.

Workforce

Healthcare is a service industry and for many, the NHS is inseparable from the staff who work in it. However, the NHS workforce is exceptional not just because of the respect it commands – other special features make workforce planning a critical function in the NHS including:

- It perhaps goes without saying, but delivering health services needs staff. Often, it also needs very specific staff: specialisation across diseases, locations of care, severity of illness have all led to a patchwork of professions and skills. There is sometimes an ability to substitute one type of workforce for another, but `generalism' is relatively rare. This means new services, or rapid expansions of old ones, can quickly run into staff shortages that take years to correct; and

- Added to this, training the workforce takes time such that, largely, we know what the workforce of 2020 will look like because it is largely already here. Partly because it does take such time, it is also an expensive resource to develop. Workforce planning matters because its effects are felt for many years and is expensive to correct.

This means workforce planning is essential but not easy and needs to meld together responding to short-term pressures as well as making progress on the strategic direction. It was perhaps one of the key advantages of the 2000 NHS Plan that it took a ten-year perspective on improving NHS services and as such could plan the workforce over a relatively long time.[12] Unfortunately from the perspective of 2015, the NHS is now facing widespread workforce challenges with critical shortages of GPs and of nurses to name but two. Difficulties in recruiting permanent nursing staff has also led to a surge in more expensive temporary staffing and evolved into a financial headache for the entire NHS. As serious as these short-term issues are they must not distract the system from the longer-term strategic goal of enhanced services in community settings and parity of esteem for mental health necessary to both deliver the better services for an older population with more long-term conditions but also in overcoming longstanding inequities between mental and physical health.

However, balancing the short term and the long term has not proved easy. The NHS has long intended to invest in community and primary care, and to deliver better mental health services. However, it has proved very difficult to translate this into actual services (i.e. staff) with declining numbers of key elements of the community workforce and a failure to increase the number of general practitioners at the same rate as hospital consultants for example.[13] Given the time it takes to train staff in the NHS this will all place a brake on the speed of change down to 2020, even if delivering better care by drawing on the skills of existing staff such as pharmacists could help.[14]

So if the NHS needed a little magic to get from the reality of 2015 to a transformed future without too many years in between, perhaps top of the list for some alchemy would be the workforce. A wish list would include:

- more nurses willing to take permanent employment in NHS hospitals, thereby bringing the agency cost bill down and freeing up many organisations from the worry of staffing the wards;

- more GPs, to fill vacancies and reduce the pressure on the existing primary care workforce; and

- if we are in wish-fulfilment, the removal of all other workforce shortages at the same time.

It can be argued that more nurses, GPs and other staff would help the existing NHS work as it is supposed to, but of course GPs are also pivotal in delivering the future with its enhanced services in primary and community settings as well. However, looking to the future models of care, we could also wish for:

- a strategic shift in the balance of the workforce and its skills: raising the capacity and capability of those working in community settings (even if their employer remained the acute hospital) and doing the same for mental health; and

- matching the policy integration with social care, the VCS and wider public health functions by achieving a greater integration of the workforce actually delivering health and care. This would mean, for example, routinely considering the capability and capacity available in the VCS when considering the local workforce and its assets.

In the absence of magic, policymakers need to be able to plan from the workforce of 2015 down to that for 2020 and 2030: given NHS employers (for example) requested declining numbers of mental health nurses down to 2020, such a plan is still work in progress.

Conclusion

The NHS has huge strengths. It has the support of the public of England (and indeed, the voters of the entire UK) in a way few other countries can boast. It has a talented and dedicated workforce. To meet the demands of a changing population it has recognised the need to change and is developing plans to do so – it is no mean feat to have brought so many stakeholders together in agreement over long-term strategy. The clouds look much darker in the immediate months and years and certainly the NHS faces some major challenges in 2015, not least over the rapidly rising tide of deficits spreading across providers, difficulties in recruitment and declining budgets in key partners of which social care is the most critical.

If an answer can be found to these immediate challenges, then one might think that the future path – while not easy – is at least clear. In this section I have argued that even if the plans of the Five Year Forward View can be brought about there is still scope for change. The benefits from placing the NHS and social care on a more stable, predictable financial footing would underpin all of its long-term planning. The need for greater integration with social care that includes financial integration, and the benefits of closer working with the other key levers that influence our health and wellbeing, offer opportunities that the NHS working alone cannot unlock. Lastly, while re-structuring the NHS workforce is not possible quickly, we need to make progress in achieving the strategic shift in our workforce that underpins the wider strategy to improve community-based services and mental health. It will not be possible to do the latter without doing the former.

Public health policy and practice: facing the future

David J. Hunter

Public health faces major challenges in a political context that, in England at any rate, is largely unfavourable to government-led intervention and which is seeking to redefine the public realm by shrinking the state. At the same time, there is growing recognition that the 'wicked' problems public health wrestles with, such as obesity, smoking, alcohol misuse and mental health, are central to the future and financial sustainability of the NHS since the growing demands on it largely derive from lifestyle related diseases which are avoidable and preventable. The NHS chief executive, Simon Stevens, in contrast to most of his predecessors has put public health and prevention high on his list of priorities for transforming the health system.

We know public health works because, globally, life expectancy doubled during the twentieth century largely as a result of reductions in child mortality which are attributable to public health measures including immunisation coverage, clean water, sanitation and other measures.[1] Chronic diseases kill twice as many people as infectious diseases. We also know, as the government's adviser, Derek Wanless, pointed out over

10 years ago, that healthier populations are more productive and economically viable ones.[2] It should be a truism that everyone benefits if people are healthy but in reality the issues are more complex and riven with powerful vested interests. The recent fracas in England over the pros and cons of a sugar tax, with celebrity chef Jamie Oliver leading the campaign in favour of a tax, is a case in point. Like health policy more generally, public health is an intensely political business.

To bring about change requires getting serious about prevention and engaging directly with the political context with the aim of reshaping and redirecting policy. But in the redesign of health systems that is under way in many countries, including the UK, public health has a key role although it is one that remains to be fully realised. This chapter endeavours to set out the nature of the challenge and reviews the prospects of it being met including how public health has to reposition itself if it is to succeed.

The present state of public health

Before we can sensibly consider how to reposition public health to give it greater prominence in a redesigned health system, a goal that has eluded successive governments, we need to understand where it has been and where it now figures in public policy in order both to decide what is worth preserving in the present arrangements and also why some elements may no longer be fit for purpose, if they ever were.

It is a time of unprecedented change and challenge for those working in public health and for those concerned about its future direction and impact. What we mean by the term 'public' is possibly more uncertain than at any other time in its history as a consequence of the shifting boundary that is under way between the state and the individual in line with government policy aimed at shrinking and redefining the state. One significant outcome of such a strategy is the transfer of greater responsibility to the individual which then leads to a focus on behaviour change as the primary means of improving health and wellbeing. It should be stated at the outset that such a direction is not immutable or unavoidable or the only option available – it is a matter of political choice. Those who assert 'there is no other way' are wrong or disingenuous or both. In politics there is always another way – it is a matter of values and choice. Politics is about who gets what, where and how. We ignore that reality at our peril.

But if we remain unclear about what the term 'public' means, especially in a health context, then similarly what we mean by terms like the 'public realm' or the 'public interest' is also less clear than might have been the case even a decade or so ago. In the shift from a welfare to a market state such notions appear to be clear-cut and well understood when it comes to defence and security issues but they become distinctly fuzzier and increasingly problematic where social and health or welfare policies are concerned.[3] If nothing else, it might be argued, public health is all about the public in some shape or form. Otherwise it is meaningless. Therein lies the tension. If what we understand by the term 'the public' is looking decidedly less obvious and fragile then where does this leave what is commonly referred to as the public health function?

Unpacking the public health function

A key distinction lies in regard to whether we view the public as a collection of individuals or as constituting something greater than the sum of its parts, that is, something more akin to a community of interest. If the focus is on self-seeking individuals then public health is likely to centre its efforts on individual behaviour change, possibly by altering the incentive structure (or what behavioural economists refer to as the 'choice architecture') facing individuals as they make decisions affecting their health.

But if we view the public as a community of interest or as occupying places and spaces, then the focus of attention shifts to the social or structural determinants of health and the factors contributing to these. Of course, in practice, public health embraces both perspectives since tackling a 'wicked problem' like obesity involves multiple approaches rather than there being a single or simple solution. The famous spaghetti diagram of the causes of obesity from the 2007 Foresight report showed graphically that environmental solutions at a macro level were required alongside those focusing on individuals at the micro level with lots of other interventions being required at various levels in between.[4] Only then would we stand a chance of combating the causes of obesity. And that call has resurfaced in McKinsey's global health report on obesity[5] and in NHS England's Five Year Forward View.[6]

Arguably, between 1974 and 2013, public health lost its way in England. Being part of the NHS, as it was during this period, proved to be a mixed blessing because the focus on individuals, ill health and on healthcare as distinct from health and wellbeing proved overwhelming. Returning public health to local government in England in 2013 heralded the prospect of a more balanced approach and one where the emphasis on place and community was positively encouraged. Apart from those wedded to a largely medical model of public health, many working in public health welcomed the move back to local government since it offered a fresh opportunity to think about health and wellbeing in a more holistic sense and address many of the root causes of health and inequality set out in the Marmot review.[7]

However, the transition from the NHS to local government has not been without its difficulties and challenges.[8] Perhaps the major one takes us back to the issue of the shrinking state and the place of the public in it. Whether one agrees with the policy or not, local government is being required to sustain among the deepest and most extensive public spending cuts and many of the worst affected local authorities are those in the most deprived areas where needs are greatest. For public health, some believe it is the perfect storm. As long as public health sat within the NHS, and notwithstanding the occasional budget raid, it seemed reasonably safe from incurring severe budget cuts. That is no longer the case in the harsher world of deep local government spending cuts and while public health may have had a degree of protection through the ring-fenced budget, that will not survive beyond the present year. Nor did it stop the chancellor from inflicting a surprising cut of £200 million on the public health budget in 2015 soon after the general election.

New directions for public health

While there is every reason to be despondent about public health and its uncertain future, not all is doom and gloom – or need not be. There are other developments occurring which could lead to a renaissance of local government and its place in the governance for health. Following Devo Manc and the

Northern Powerhouse initiative, local government is back centre stage with an opportunity to reinvent itself. The issue is whether it can do so when the context in which it is operating could not be less propitious or more unforgiving. Given the position of retrenchment in which it finds itself, in terms of resources and services, it becomes all too easy for central government to indulge in 'blame diffusion' when things go wrong, pointing the finger at local government and asserting it was simply not up to the job. Certainly there are many in local government who predict (and fear) such an outcome and who will not rush into embracing healthcare as a devolved function until they see what the likely risks are.

And there are many possible risks if local government takes a keener interest in health, including healthcare. As long as it was only responsible for public health separate from other parts of healthcare then there was some hope that it would come out from under the shadows of acute hospital care where it had been hiding for most of the 40 or so years from 1974. But if part of the devolution settlement is for local government to take on responsibility for healthcare services, albeit within agreed guidelines to ensure that the 'national' remains within the NHS, there has to be a risk that public health will once again be sidelined as the urgent forever drives out the important. Hospital closures bring people out onto the streets. Terminating smoking cessation services does not.

The paradox of all this is that just at a time when public health could be undergoing a renaissance following its shift back to local government, it may prove short-lived if a more general oversight of the NHS across a local community absorbs all the attention and available resources. We would then be back where we started unless local authorities are able to exercise vigilance over their public health responsibilities. However it is by no means self-evident that all elected members would see it as being in their interests to put public health first when faced with addressing immediate pressures arising from the state of the NHS in their communities.

It is just possible that such a fate may be avoided as a result of another paradox occurring simultaneously. The generally highly praised and widely endorsed NHS Five Year Forward View has in effect become the government's de facto health policy.[9] But unlike any previous such policy, it makes a big play on the need for the NHS to take public health seriously and to become a staunch advocate for it at all levels and through a variety of means, some of which mean taking on big business, including the powerful big food and drink companies.

What a supreme irony. No sooner has public health been removed from the NHS than the NHS is being berated for ignoring it and cajoled to do more to promote it. This is not pink fluffy stuff. The hard-nosed argument underpinning the NHS chief executive's personal exhortation is that neither the NHS, nor any health system anywhere relying on public funding, is sustainable in the face of rising levels of illness caused by lifestyle factors, notably obesity, which are essentially avoidable. But the issues go further since an unhealthy population is an economic drag in other ways too as well as contributing to widening health inequalities.

It was a banker (though before it became a term of opprobrium), Derek Wanless, who in 2002 published his report setting out the challenges facing the NHS up to 2022 and the policy response needed. He criticised the

NHS for being a sickness rather than a health service and argued persuasively that unless urgent action was taken to reverse this approach, the NHS would become unaffordable. It would seem he was right. Although he said little that was new and which the public health community had not been articulating for many years, the fact that it was a respected businessman making the case registered with government. They accepted his analysis and recommendations even if progress in implementing them has been faltering at best.

Over a decade later, the Five Year Forward View takes up the same challenge, having criticised both central government and the NHS for failing to heed Wanless's warning. He lamented the lack of robust evidence concerning interventions and their effectiveness or otherwise and the reasons for failure. Nor was he exercised about which interventions should be the focus of attention. The key issue for him was whether they worked or not and, if not, why not. A similar approach informs the Five Year Forward View which calls for action at all levels including taxing unhealthy food products (eg sugar), and reformulating food to reduce high levels of salt and sugar. But these are actions that only government can take especially if change at a population level is going to happen. The arguments are convincingly set out in Public Health England's report on sugar, calling for action at all levels, from the individual to government.[10]

The problem is that for governments of all persuasions, perhaps especially those in thrall to vested interests, there is a deep seated resistance to taking action which seeks to tackle the structural and social causes of poor public health. It is much simpler and neatly sidesteps the 'nanny state' charge if government policy is restricted to providing information to the public on how to lead healthier lives. Tackling the root causes of ill health can be put to one side on the grounds that intervening would be seen as meddling in people's lives and restricting their freedom of choice.

This tension between government action at a societal level to tackle public health challenges on the one hand and, on the other, action focused on individual lifestyle behaviour change, runs through public health like a fault line. It has been termed 'lifestyle drift' to reflect the tendency of governments, even those seemingly well-disposed to population wide interventions, to resort to actions confined to lifestyle change through education, providing information and nudging behaviour in favour of healthier lifestyles.[11] Yet the evidence that such an approach can work or work at a scale and pace required to make a significant difference is weak and unconvincing. Such policies need to be part of the mix to tackle a complex public health issue like obesity but they can never be the whole or sole answer. A well-crafted policy response demands other measures and these tend to be those which only government action can sanction.

Apart from wishing to steer clear of the nanny state charge, governments struggle for other reasons to make progress in tackling stubborn and deep-seated health problems. For the most part public policy functions are compartmentalised and located in a variety of departmental silos which invariably display tribal behaviours that are not conducive to collaborative working and joining up functions across government. Yet an effective response to many public health challenges demands a whole of government approach in which there is good alignment between the different parts of government that may have an impact on health and wellbeing. The Finnish government's Health in All Policies (HiAP) initiative recognises such concerns[12] and the World Health Organization HiAP training manual endeavours to equip policymakers and practitioners with the requisite skills.[13]

The revolution in healthcare which the secretary of state for health, Jeremy Hunt, says is upon us will put the patient at the centre of his or her healthcare, making a reality of the joke 'the patient will see you now'. But this revolution risks focusing further on an individualistic view of health, thereby reinforcing lifestyle drift in policy.

Building on community assets

To ensure that population health remains high on the policy agenda, a different revolution is required. This would mobilise and empower communities and galvanise public opinion to influence and shape public policy. Whole of society approaches, perhaps adopting asset based thinking to work with the grain of communities, lie at the heart of this effort. It has been described as the third era in health (the first era focusing on medical care and the second era focusing on the healthcare system) and one which focuses on creating the capacities to achieve goals for equitable health improvement through community-integrated health systems focusing on population health goals.[14] There would be an emphasis on health outcomes for geographically defined populations, including on upstream socioeconomic factors that influence health. The role of those working in public health would be to enable and nurture community integrated health systems working with local groups to reduce community risk factors and provide coordinated support to strengthen health and wellbeing.

Adopting such an approach will require viewing the creation and maintenance of health as a form of co-production between public health practitioners and local communities. Working together they will become co-designers of healthy communities and the behaviours required within them to ensure and sustain health. Those communities would also become better informed and equipped to be more effective advocates for improved health.

Such an approach ties in neatly with the newfound emphasis on devolution epitomised by the government's Northern Powerhouse initiative noted earlier. In those areas, like Greater Manchester, where local government is assuming responsibility for healthcare there will be a real opportunity to reengineer what currently exists into a third era health system. Of course there are risks, as mentioned earlier, notably that local government will find itself unable to adopt a whole system perspective or become captured by the vested interests within the existing healthcare system who are seeking to maintain their resources and services even where these have been shown to be ineffective and not fit for purpose. Such dynamics and outcomes may be appropriate for second era healthcare but not for third era health system thinking that is concerned with the whole system of which healthcare is a part in the effort, to optimise health.

These developments to rethink the role of the state in health and move towards a third era health system align well with the notion of the 'relational state' which offers a critique of both traditional bureaucratic public services and market-based approaches. Instead, it seeks to find a new alliance between government and governed.[15] The relational state eschews both bureaucratic and market forces in favour of human relationships. Whereas the state can be remote from, and insensitive to, community needs and preferences, markets tend to commodify relationships that should not be commodified. Such thinking has profound implications for the future shape of the public health workforce and the skills it will need to function in a relational state.

Rethinking the public health workforce

Working with and through communities will require a necessary shift in mindset on the part of public health practitioners and those who lead them. Coupled with the significant resource pressures on public health, which are unlikely to ease up or be reversed any time soon, the matter of what the public health workforce is for and who comprises it becomes an interesting and critical issue. Indeed, it is one receiving attention from the Royal Society of Public Health and by the Department of Health backed People in the UK Public Health (PIUKPH) group, which is advising the UK health departments on an overarching strategy for the public health workforce with the goal of improving the public's health. The group's starting point is a recognition that improving the public's health involves a broad range of people in a variety of professions, communities and settings.

Changes in the workforce seem desirable if not essential for several reasons, some positive and others arguably less so. At a time of spending cuts and retrenchment, it makes sense to harness and put to good use already existing skills many of which may be found in those roles and occupations who may not regard themselves as doing public health or as public health practitioners but whose actions nevertheless impact on the public's health. This is the view of PIUKPH who include in the wider public health workforce not only familiar services such as community pharmacy and the fire and police but also postal workers, librarians, leisure staff, hairdressers and cleaners. The wider workforce is defined as 'any individual who is not a specialist or practitioner in public health, but has the opportunity or ability to positively impact health and wellbeing through their (paid or unpaid) work'.[16] The headcount for the wider workforce is 20.2 million people, comprised of 57 occupational groups.

But whatever the future holds for the workforce, even within traditional public health practice there is a need for new and different skills to meet contemporary challenges brought about by social, technological and other changes. In the digital age focused on individual lifestyles and health monitoring, how can a balance be achieved so that the wider determinants of health are not ignored or overlooked. The skill base to meet this challenge does not lie in epidemiology but in the ability to exhibit and exercise 'soft power' skills centred on relationship building, negotiation, conflict management, political astuteness, communication and presentation. Leadership style is also critical and one that no longer adheres to the 'great man' theory of leadership but rather is concerned with developing leadership that attempts to be more inclusive and adaptive to particular contexts. We also require leaders who are able to pose the right questions and bring together those best able and placed to explore solutions to them rather than expecting leaders to have all the answers. In the case of those 'wicked issues' with which public health perennially wrestles, there are no easy, simple or single solutions.

But, given what was discussed above, we also require leaders who can engage with the public and seek their input into how to improve community health and wellbeing. For too long, public health has excluded the public and focused instead on government, industry and individuals. These stakeholders are important and remain key to any effective policy intervention but, as Wanless pointed out over a decade ago when he devised his 'fully engaged' scenario, a key component of this must be that 'levels of public engagement in relation to their health are high'.[17] To achieve this requires mobilising public opinion so that the public becomes a firm ally in efforts to combat those forces antagonistic to health and wellbeing.

Conclusion

We know that public scepticism with existing political parties and the political system as a whole is at an all-time high. The widespread perception exists that governments do not reflect the public interest but rather the interests of their corporate donors. If public health is to have a future and be a vigorous force for change, then it needs to be at the forefront of a new politics aimed at mobilising public opinion and engaging the public in the improvement of population health and wellbeing. Such a task goes beyond individual behaviour change based on nudge thinking and requires support from the state as an enabler of the new relationships that need to be created, both horizontally and vertically within government and society.

Can decentralisation and personal responsibility help re-structure the NHS?

Richard B. Saltman

That stability is one of the most important characteristics of a hospital and of a healthcare system is widely agreed by physicians, patients, and politicians alike. As the well-known business school maxim puts it, when medical staff come in to work on Monday morning, they should know exactly what they are supposed to do. While perhaps not as famous as Aneurin Bevan's centralist political demand that 'if a hospital bedpan is dropped in a hospital corridor in Tredegar, the reverberations should echo around Whitehall', in practice it is the day-to-day operational dimensions of healthcare institutions that determine the quality of care they provide, the efficacy of the clinical outcomes they achieve, and the long-term credibility of the institutions they run. Put simply, institutional stability is a necessary objective of both good policy and good management in the health sector.

The problem with stability, however, is that it always comes hand in hand with an ugly twin, stasis. Stasis is the visible face of organisational rigidity, of clinical backwardness, of antiquated work rules and oppressive bureaucratic oversight. Just as stability is essential and prized, stasis is corrosive and destructive. Yet in every large work organisation – especially in publicly operated and controlled provider organisations like hospitals – stability and stasis seem to be two sides of the same structural coin.

This core operational quandary afflicts both policy and management in publicly operated healthcare systems. And it is this core quandary that publicly run health systems have such difficulty in addressing. If one looks back over both the policy and management literature during the last 30 years, one can find numerous examples of 'magic bullets' that have been hailed as solutions to this stability-stasis problem. Among the better known in the policy world have been Deming's, then Donabedian's, then Don Berwick's quality assurance mechanisms; Fetter and Thompson's Diagnostic-Related Groups case-based payment framework;[1] primary care control – via doctor/clinic/board/group practice – over hospital budgets via various forms of contracting mechanisms; and today's current favorites: value-based payment systems, lean six sigma management, payment for performance, and patient safety assurance programs (eg 'never events', etc).

All of these proposed strategies have had some success. Many of them continue in some form in different parts of most tax-funded healthcare systems. Yet all of them have had a relatively short half-life to their magic bullet status, and most have now faded into just one more aspect of a still difficult struggle to prioritise management stability combined with high standard clinical outcomes.

The above perspective is not intended to argue that all healthcare reform in a publicly operated system like the NHS is futile. Indeed, as just stated, many of the above strategies have made valuable incremental improvements. Conversely, it also isn't to agree with public sector apologists who pretend that all is perfectly fine with existing tax-funded healthcare systems if politicians would simply find the courage (or integrity, in some versions) to just dramatically raise taxes on 'the rich'.

Of the multiple solutions pursued to date, however, it should be noted that most have also added considerably to organisational complexity, and, conversely, that few have changed the fundamental reality that stability still comes hand-in-hand with stasis. Moreover, in England as elsewhere in northern (and southern) Europe, one can hear a continued outcry about institutional fixedness and the consequent harm to patient care and sometimes patient survival in healthcare debates in 2015 much as one heard in 1983 (the general manager reform), in 1989 (the efficiency trap debate), in 1997 (the contestability vs. competition debate), in 2003 (the central regulation vs. semi-autonomous trust management debate) and in 2010 (the commissioning vs. bureaucracy debate).

This long-running discussion of the inability of past health reform strategies to resolve the stability-stasis institutional logjam raises the obvious question of what new strategy, what new measures can break the thirty year old logjam? What structural or managerial change might work better, and why?

An equally important dilemma that weighs on this assessment: the apparent end of substantial long-term economic growth in Europe, and with it the end of substantial new revenues for what are increasingly more expensive healthcare services.[2][3][4] That the UK, like Germany, at this writing is currently generating a small positive level of growth – under 3% – does not appreciably alter the dire long-term scenario. The UK has an extraordinary amount of public debt piled up since the onset of the 2008 financial crisis, which continues to grow. Britain's Office for National Statistics reported on 22 September 2015 that borrowing for deficit spending had again jumped in August 2015[5] and that government departmental spending had also jumped – a widening of an already 3.7% planned annual deficit for fiscal 2015-2016 that must be added to an unsustainable national debt which runs to over 90% of GDP. Further, the British Office for National Statistics reported on September 19, 2015 that overall labour productivity in 2014 in the UK had fallen to a full 30% lower than that of France, Germany and the United States – setting the stage for greater difficulty in paying down the UK's sovereign debt as well as for considerably lower living standards in England in the future. Chancellor George Osborne concluded two months earlier, in July, that raising productivity was 'the challenge of our lifetime'.[6]

Readers also may find it surprising to learn that emerging market countries – particularly the BRIC countries (Brazil, Russia, India and China) – now produce a larger proportion of the world economy than does all of the European Union, the United States, Japan, Canada, and the Antipodes combined.[7] This suggests the scope of the economic challenge that developed countries like the UK face in finding new revenues for social spending like health services. As Stephen D. King, previously chief economist at HSBC Bank, has framed this broader policy quandary:

'Our disturbing early twenty-first century reality of stagnation cannot be so easily ignored... Without reasonable growth, we cannot meet the entitlements we created for ourselves. These promises can only be met... if our economies continue to expand at a rate we have become accustomed to. Stagnation chips away at our entitlements, bit by bit.'[8]

Thus the NHS, like most other tax-funded healthcare systems, finds itself facing very un-Bevanite structural decisions about developing new, more diverse provider arrangements which can operate with more stability but less stasis in a climate of ever scarcer financial resources.[9] Further, serious questions can be raised about the need to identify additional, non-public sources of revenue.[10]

There have been a raft of reports coming out from England in the last year or so that arrive (gingerly) at one or both of these uncomfortable policy conclusions. These include King's Fund's 'A New Settlement' (2014) and John Appleby's 50-year projection of what funding the NHS will not have);[11] Julian Le Grand's 2014 report from the UK Cabinet Office on the potential future role of not-for-profit private providers;[12] the Dalton Report's reluctant conclusion that more private providers will be required,[13] and the NHS Executive's own conclusions about the healthcare service's fiscal distress in its Five Year Forward View.[14]

As a contribution to this ongoing debate about future strategies for the English NHS, this chapter will examine two structural reform proposals sometimes put forward as potential new 'magic bullets'. One is decentralisation of governance inside the NHS, particularly the idea of combining health and social care under local governments. The second is increased personal responsibility, on the service production side through self-care and self-monitoring, and/or on the financing side through the use of greater out-of-pocket payments as well as both positive and negative financial incentives tied to health-related behaviour.

Both decentralisation and personal responsibility trigger the same broad policy questions. First, can some form of either or both of these two strategies help reduce stasis and organisational rigidity, generating better quality of care and better value for money? Second, can they help the NHS survive financially in an era of slow economic growth? Third, in the pursuit of efficiency, do they risk damaging equity of access (either by social class or by geography) and/or equity of clinical outcomes? In short, can either decentralisation and personal responsibility – or some combination – generate sufficient change to become a new 'silver bullet' that can help re-vitalise the existing structure of service?

Decentralisation

Decentralisation has recently come back on the British policy agenda as a potential strategy to help the English NHS deal with its fiscal and structural difficulties. As part of the current Conservative government's initiative to find less administratively expensive operating models for the public sector, a major pilot will begin operation in Greater Manchester, where a regionally elected mayor and council will take responsibility for a £7 billion budget and all locally provided health as well as social services.[15]

There already is a substantial range of de facto decentralisation built into existing NHS administrative arrangements inside England. Most public hospitals are now managed as foundation trusts with considerable local managerial autonomy. Many local commissioning groups have contracts for services with private NFP and FP providers. Public-private partnerships (PPPs) have contracted private companies to build and lease back new hospitals to local trusts. All of these elements are part of a New Public Management approach that has been introduced into NHS operations over the past 20 years.

Thus further efforts with this type of administrative or internal decentralisation would not represent a new departure. What then is different about the type of decentralisation that will be introduced in Manchester, and which some propose as a potential strategy for the NHS across the entire country?

In England as elsewhere, there seem to be almost as many definitions of decentralisation as there are proponents. Everyone has their own idea of what a well-functioning re-distribution of authority downward to smaller entities – which is what decentralisation consists of – should look like. Moreover, since decentralisation is a political concept being applied in a political arena, it inevitably gets re-shaped by historical, geographical, demographic and cultural demands as well as by the immediate political needs of those putting it into place. Not surprisingly, seemingly similar decentralisation proposals often differ considerably when examined more closely.

The most widely cited formal definition is that of Rondinelli (1981) who split decentralisation into four different structural sub-types:

- *deconcentration* – national policy and/or management decisions but administered by lower level, regional or district offices staffed by nationally appointed, managed and paid staff.

- *devolution* – lower level region or district makes policy and/or management decisions, sometimes on a constitutionally mandated and protected basis, typically within a broad policy framework that is nationally determined but administered by locally elected officials (Scottish, Welsh, and Northern Irish control over health services falls under this category).

- *delegation* – specific regulatory or supervisory responsibilities are farmed out to private sector non-profit organisations (eg the British Medical Association to discipline physician behavior) and/or private for-profit organisations (health insurers in The Netherlands).

- *privatisation* – selling publicly owned hospitals, health centers, ambulance services, etc, to a new private sector owner.

All four of these structural sub-types of decentralisation involve a reduction of the national government's direct control over decision-making, however the government typically retains a steering role in shaping the landscape, setting boundary conditions regarding performance, and retaining the inevitable political possibility of clawing back the authority it had given away. Thus whichever basic form of decentralisation is introduced, the ensuing process always involves a constantly adjusting balance of decision-making authority – often both formal and implicit – between national and non-national decision-makers.

Beyond these four structural types of decentralisation, in practice decentralisation also has three core functional dimensions: political/policy-making, administrative/operational, and fiscal.[16] These three functions operate more-or-less independently, and thus one or two can be partly or completely decentralised at the same time that the remaining function(s) can continue to be fully centralised.

In the Swedish healthcare system, as one example, political decision-making is shared out between national and regional/county governments, while administrative responsibilities have been almost completely decentralised to the regional/county level (although the national government still plays a strong regulatory role over quality, safety, annual co-payment ceilings, and other standards of service, as well as pharmaceutical approvals and bulk purchases through the state-owned company Apotekbolaget). Further, while fiscal decision-making is mostly a regional/county responsibility, the national government can apply certain limits to regional/county taxation rates (as was done in the early 1990s to stabilise overall public expenditures in the run-up to EU admission in 1995) and often makes targeted grants to regions/counties to ensure equity of services across rural and metropolitan parts of the country as well as to stimulate new or lagging clinical activities and also to encourage consolidation of some highly specialised services among regions.[17]

The reasons why governments choose to decentralise are myriad and complex. Ultimately, however, they derive from two specific policy expectations. One can be termed the 'democratic argument' – that a decentralised health system structure is 'closer to the people' (devolution, deconcentration) and thus will provide services that are a better fit to local needs and preferences. The second is a variety of different, sometimes contradictory, 'economic arguments' about improving efficiency and/or fostering quality and cost competition between local governmental units.[18]

As this Swedish example highlights, decentralisation in the contemporary political world is hardly ever a unitary all-or-nothing decision. Rather, parts of various functions, decisions, and responsibilities are typically split between the several parties to a decentralised governance structure. The result is a type of counterbalance, in which one party to a decentralisation process – whether national or non-national – can only go so far before the other involved parties will need to accommodate and accept any proposed changes. Some analysts see this as positive restraint on overweening governmental authority, in keeping with the balance of power approach of political philosophers like the 17th Century French Montesquieu and American founding fathers Thomas Jefferson and James Madison. Others seethe at what they contend is the bureaucratic inefficiency of multiple decision-makers and, they claim, the resulting weak and incremental decision-making process.

A key policy issue inherent in all four forms of decentralisation is that, because none of them is unitary in structure, the results from a partly or fully decentralised health system also are normally not unitary. Thus the advantages of a decentralised system, in which some local units deliver care in a different manner than other units, inexorably result in some local units having better or worse outcomes than other units. This difference in outcomes has become an important political issue in strongly decentralised healthcare systems such as in Finland and Sweden, where proponents of equality not only of access but of outcomes argue sharply that care is 'unequal' and thus unfair despite formal legal protections (as in Sweden).

Yet the entire point of introducing decentralisation is to free up local decision-making on one or more of the three functional dimensions of decentralisation, precisely so that each one is able to make different decisions than their neighboring unit, based either on a different set of local preferences, or a different strategy to utilise economic pressures to improve overall operating and cost efficiencies. Thus decentralisation, if it is working properly, *should* produce different outcomes for different types of patients, at least until more effective strategies can be spread more widely through a focus on best practices. And while this emphasis on differential outcomes need not resemble the class-based differences traditionally associated with post-code rationing, different districts will perform differently. Moreover, these different local decisions may affect outcomes: there is some evidence now in Sweden that some cancer patients are moving their entire household from one region/county into another in order to gain higher priority for life-saving but expensive new drugs.[19]

In sum, decentralisation comes in a range of different formats, all of which can be seen as having their advantages as well as their disadvantages depending on one's interests and perspective.[20][21] The upshot here, from a practical policy point of view, is that it is a supremely flexible policy tool that can be adopted by decision-makers as they find politically useful. There is no right or wrong point of view about the structure or impact of decentralisation. Quite differently, its usefulness is conditional: it depends on the context within which it is being proposed, as that context determines how much gets decentralised, to who/whom, at what potential benefit and with what potential costs. Thus every decision about decentralisation involves a balancing of factors and outcomes, such that what is appropriate in one context may well not be in another, making policy modelling difficult.

Personal responsibility

The notion of personal responsibility is anathema to most defenders of the traditional English NHS. Nothing creates more ideological apoplexy (likely on view in one or two adjacent chapters in this book) than suggestions that individual citizens and patients should be required to contribute directly to their healthcare either medically or financially. Such proposals are immediately attacked as violations of the core principles of solidarity and equality that defenders argue have undergirded the NHS since its inception (for a more realistic view of the shifting content of solidarity in health systems over time, see Saltman 2015).[22]

This fundamental aversion is a bit curious, however, given that the language of the 2009 NHS Constitution's section 2b, 'Patients and the public – your responsibilities,' includes the indicative if weakly phrased statement that 'you can make a significant contribution to your own, and your family's good health, and take some responsibility for it'.[23] More practically, with regard to patient monitoring and other emerging forms of patient co-production of care, most providers know well that patients themselves take responsibility for and meet more than two-thirds of their medical needs. This is especially true for primary care services.[24]

Additionally, for frail elderly patients who require in-home custodial services, the usual estimates in developed countries are that roughly 70% of all custodial care is provided by informal caregivers, consisting of unpaid family members and neighbours and/or paid immigrants and other informal non-governmental non-professional workers. Several Nordic governments now provide a range of dedicated supports for these informal caregivers, including call-in lines and respite care, in order to encourage them to continue to keep these elderly out of expensive nursing homes.[25] [26]

With regard to patient co-production of clinical care, new techniques enable medical staff to monitor heart rates, blood sugar, and other vital signs over web-based connections, identifying problems before they result in crisis trips to the hospital. New electronic systems in the home, managed by the patient, can monitor a diabetic's blood sugar and then send instructions to an implanted insulin pump so as to maintain a steady level. Similar monitoring and intervention are being developed for a range of other chronic conditions. In the US, the Massachusetts Institute of Technology and other engineering schools conduct regular tutorials for electronically knowledgeable parents who want to 'hack' current electronic systems to enable them to better monitor and intervene in dealing with their childrens' chronic medical conditions.[27]

While self-care and self-monitoring in the production of healthcare can in some circumstances be controversial (on both patient safety and union employment grounds), the harshest arguments aimed against individual responsibility inevitably occur on the financial side, concerning efforts to increase individual out-of-pocket payments. Defenders of collective public financing already dislike existing charges which individuals must pay privately in the UK healthcare arena: some outpatient pharmaceuticals, dental care, eyeglasses, and medications or treatments outside the approved NHS formulary – this last a subject of often bitter debate for some drugs and treatments: consider as examples Herceptin[28] and Kadcyla[29]) for breast cancer, and proton radiation treatment.[30] Individuals also have to make substantial payments for nursing home and home care services beyond certain cost, savings and capital points, with some elderly required to sell their homes to help pay for that care.[31]

Out-of-pocket payments for necessary clinical services and supplies remain controversial among health policy analysts. That lower income individuals won't seek out care if they have to pay more out of pocket, despite having poor overall health status, is well documented in the academic literature.[32] Indeed a traditional function of collective rather than individual finance is to ensure that precisely this differentiation of access to care by income level is reduced to as low a level as financially feasible.

Given, however, the persistent lack of strong economic growth in the UK as in other developed economies, government decision-makers really only have two economically feasible choices about future health sector financing. One alternative is to continue exclusively public funding, which, given the inability to raise already very high tax levels, will necessarily fall farther and farther behind what is needed to maintain the rapidly increasing international standard of good clinical care, especially in treating cancers. The other alternative is to try to find the least socially damaging mechanisms to collect additional private revenue from patients and or citizens, supplemented by separate indigent relief funds.[33]

In practice, what this second alternative calls for is to shift the currently existing boundary that separates healthcare services and supplies (e.g. outpatient drugs) which are either provided entirely by public sector professionals or which are funded entirely by public sector taxes on a collective basis, and those which are only partly or not-at-all provided and/or funded collectively and which must therefore be provided and/or paid for by the patient, the client, or the individual citizen. Much as noted above regarding policy frameworks for decentralisation, the boundary that separates collective public from individual private responsibility is partial, permeable, and subject to the particular social, political and economic context in which it exists. Policy responses in this arena – especially regarding financial charges and co-payments –is almost infinitely variable depending upon the financial pressures that policymakers confront and their judgment about how much lower or higher private costs and payments can feasibly be pushed. While in earlier periods of rapid economic growth, the debate was often about moving more services out from the private and into the collective public sphere, current prolonged economic stagnation is forcing decision-makers to concentrate on which services to move in the other direction, from public to private responsibility. Numerous current examples of these boundary issues can be found in the differing responses of national governments to the 2008 fiscal crisis.[34][35]

On this topic, UK readers may find it interesting to learn that the boundaries for publicly funded care are drawn quite differently in the German social insurance system,[36] where individuals have a clear legal responsibility to maintain their health.

First, Article 1 of the Social Code Book #5 governing the German health insurance system states:

> The insured have co-responsibility for their health; through a health-conscious way of living, taking part in appropriately timed preventive measures and playing an active role in treatment and

rehabilitation, they should contribute to avoiding illness and disability...

Second, funds are allowed to give individuals financial payments of up to 100 euros for participation in different prevention measures.[37] If adults participate in annual check-up programs with no lapses for 5 years, by law the health insurance fund must pay $\frac{2}{5}$ths of the individuals' annual insurance premium – $\frac{3}{5}$ths if there are no lapses for 10 years. Also, premium deductions up to 20% are possible for those who participate in a less expensive, but narrowed network of managed care.

Moving beyond existing efforts in Germany to define the boundary between collective and individual responsibility, UK readers may also find it useful to learn about the values-based screens which German and Swedish academics have developed to test the social acceptability of various different co-payment or self-payment requirements.

In the first framework, drawing on German and US experience as well as key tenets of moral philosophy, Schmidt (2010) proposed seven substantive tests with which to assess the appropriateness of measures that would increase personal responsibility:[38]

a) Evidence rationale and feasibility – 'justified in an open and transparent manner'
b) Intrusiveness and coerciveness – 'is the extent of intrusiveness justifiable'
c) Equity – 'at what point...reasonable to reject a policy because of inequitable impact'
d) Solidarity/risk-pooling – 'if (undermining solidarity)...can the effect be justified'
e) Attributability/opportunity of choice – 'rewards based on...free and voluntary choices'

f) Affected third parties – 'effect on the relationship(s) people have'
g) Coherence – 'standards of responsibility, attributability, and blame'

A second group of academics has developed a similar set of values-based tests for increased individual out-of-pocket payments in the tax-funded structure of healthcare in Sweden – which has a funding and value base quite close to that of England and the UK.

Following an earlier ethical framework for justifying the rationing of certain types of clinical services in the Netherlands,[39] Tinghogg *et al* (2010) propose a tightly defined set of six screens or filters by which to determine which services could morally be removed from the collectively funded package and thereby left to private financing and/or individual out-of-pocket payment.[40] The six 'attributes of individual responsibility' define specific services which can legitimately be transferred:

a) It should enable individuals to value need and quality both before and after utilisation;
b) It should be directed toward individuals with a reasonable level of individual autonomy;
c) It should be associated with low levels of positive externalities;
d) It should be associated with a demand of sufficient magnitude to generate a private market;
e) It should be associated with payments affordable for most individuals;
f) It should be associated with lifestyle enhancements rather than medical necessities.

Both of these moral frameworks make assumptions about the character of the external policy context that may or may not be valid. They assume that decisions about what services are to be moved from the collective to the individual sphere of financing can each be carefully assessed separately. They assume that adequate time exists for policymakers to undertake this evaluation process before establishing new policy. They assume that the public financing structure will have sufficient funds left to fund all other necessary and needed services. However, as the studies of national policy responses to the health sector consequences of the 2008 financial crisis demonstrate, most European policymakers found themselves forced to act much more rapidly,[41] and they lacked sufficient funds to pay for all care that did not pass these morally designed screens.

A further problem with this philosophy-based approach is that a number of expensive contemporary health conditions are brought on not by bad luck or medically dangerous external environments but rather by individuals' own behaviour. Conditions including obesity, diabetes, and high blood pressure often reflect in varying degree eating fatty food, heavily sweetened sodas, salt intake, and following a sedentary lifestyle (typically in front of some electronic entertainment device).

In turn, rather than relying on morally-based regulations as suggested by Schmidt and Tinghogg *et al.*, many economists would argue that the best way to obtain the necessary individual change in behaviour would be to create a monetary incentive to do so. In this view, for conditions caused primarily by poor individual choices, it may make sense to create some personal financial responsibility for making good choices.

In the US, where private companies bear much of the cost of paying for their employees healthcare services, many of those companies – as well as NFP institutions like the author's originally church-run university – now take financially focussed steps to reinforce the message that individuals need to take preventive care of their own health, so as not to cause the collective purse unnecessary costs. These typically are a mix of both positive and negative incentives. Positive incentives at the author's university – for all staff regardless of income or status – include a $200 credit on their health insurance costs if they attend an on-campus assessment of their cholesterol level, blood pressure and weight. Negative incentives – assessed simultaneously with the positive incentives – include a $600/year charge if the employee smokes cigarettes, and another $600 charge if their spouse or partner does so. These fines are foregone if the individual enters into a (free) stop-smoking course provided by the employer. It should be noted that although whether an employee smokes is self-reported, those found to lie about their smoking are subject to immediate dismissal from employment (lying by employees is viewed as dangerous to the safety of everyone else in the workplace).

To raise the possibility that charging individuals for smoking or other bad health choices should be introduced in a public tax-based system raises both moral and practical concerns. Morally, there is no doubt that lower income individuals would pay proportionately more. Practically, there would be privacy concerns about state tax charges based on individual behaviour (e.g. smoking). Moreover, it's hard to design a penalty payment structure for bad eating choices. Nonetheless, the overall contribution of poor individual choices to poor health, combined with the ceiling on publicly raised funds that many tax-funded health systems – including the NHS in England – have now clearly reached –

suggests that such penalty charges and co-payments will become increasingly politically attractive.

Overall, personal responsibility represents a policy arena that is not only politically controversial, but which can be expected to become increasingly politically attractive. As public resources fade, as public care providers are increasingly overburdened, a growing role for patient co-production and self-monitoring as well as for individual negative and positive financial incentives, carefully delimited, seems more and more likely.

Potential implications for the NHS

So what does all this academic argumentation add up to in terms of how to resolve the service delivery and funding problems that the English NHS now confronts? Can some form of decentralisation and of personal responsibility help optimise operations and outcomes from a giant public healthcare system that is slowly being unpicked by equally large and seemingly inexorable structural pressures? Can either force NHS hospitals to overcome stasis to create a more outcomes-based organisational climate?

The first response is to note that both decentralisation and personal responsibility come in many forms. The concept alone is not sufficient to achieve positive change. Instead, improvement will be contingent on how each concept is shaped, shaded, introduced, regulated, and supported – in short, on the politics of its implementation and management.

Second, since each of these two policy mechanisms brings both advantages and disadvantages, which often arrive together in the same outcome from any one specific action, again, the successful introduction of either mechanism will depend on how it is structured, and also on who is assessing that outcome.

Overall, decentralisation might well generate better targeted and more locally appropriate services, also somewhat more managerially efficient services. Assuming medical staff have local contracts to local authorities, and hence feel the importance of being responsive to local individuals and conditions, patients will likely feel better served.

However there will inevitably be duplication of function and personnel across different districts, thus decentralisation probably won't save as much money as some anticipate. Indeed, Finland, which has the most extreme decentralisation in a Western European health system, is currently struggling in the face of a protracted recession to consolidate its small municipalities into larger units so as to reduce what the national government argues are the unnecessary costs of personnel and service duplication.[42]

There also would be different medical and service outcomes in different local districts. As noted previously, there could be some convergence over time in this regard through national oversight and also the dissemination of best practice. However, for decentralisation to become accepted practice, there will have to be greater political tolerance of variation in access times, treatment options and perhaps clinical outcomes than currently.

It also should be noted that decentralisation would create additional administrative and managerial challenges. Efforts to combine social and health services under one locally operated service involves consolidation as well as decentralisation. Moreover, housing ambulatory chronic and elderly care services under the same administrative roof will not resolve the professional and organisational tensions that typically appear when physicians and social workers – two quite different professions – are expected to cooperate closely.

Turning to personal responsibility, evaluation of its impact in tax-funded health systems in Northern Europe is still quite limited. On the patient co-production and self-monitoring side, if implemented in a skilled manner into the managerial structure of NHS specialist services, personal responsibility would likely have the potential to increase the quality of care and improve patient outcomes at the same time (among many assessments see Coulter 2011).[43] It also should logically have the potential to save considerable sums by reducing overall demand from chronically ill patients for outpatient, inpatient, and emergency room visits. However these savings can only materialise if unnecessary medical staff can in fact be moved or made redundant, and if both can be done without incurring large additional administrative costs. In Sweden, as a contrary example, dismissals of publicly employed health sector staff are managerially time-consuming and financially expensive: one month salary for each year of employment must be paid as severance by law, making hospital savings through staff reduction substantially harder to achieve.

Turning to the financial dimensions of personal responsibility, here the potential health and fiscal benefits as well as the potential difficulties would both seem to be greater. The financial savings to the NHS by targeting higher co-payments on peripheral services – perhaps in keeping with the Schmidt or Tinghogg frameworks – could be quite substantial in a large service like NHS England. Further, the introduction of negative as well as positive financial incentives for health-enhancing and/or health-harming behaviour would likely improve immediate as well as longer term health benefits for individual patients and citizens, and could over a five or ten year period even begin to have an impact on overall population health statistics.

Lastly, regarding stability versus stasis, both decentralisation and personal responsibility have the potential to strengthen innovative managerial mechanisms and strategies that can erode the forces of organisational stasis and resistance. Results will depend again on the degree to which personnel unions are required to become more flexible, particularly regarding work rules as well as individual and team performance incentives. See for example the difficulties incurred in this regard by attempts to introduce more performance-oriented management by the provincial government of Valencia in Hospital de la Ribera in Alzira.[44]

One additional point: decentralisation itself can be a bit rocky to implement, especially if there are dissenting political views inside the new local governance structure, or if there is labour resistance. Thus, the advantage of decentralisation in this regard may be more that it shakes off some of the current bureaucratic stasis than that it is a guarantee of consistent operational stability across every institution and organisation.

Taken overall, the above assessment suggests that, if introduced together and in full force, decentralisation and personal responsibility could have a noticeably positive impact on how the NHS operates. Some clinical services would likely improve, and some patients may feel more confident in the quality of care they receive.

At the same time, however, it should be clear from the various caveats noted above that these mechanisms are in and of themselves not sufficient to resolve the fundamental structural and financial challenges that the

NHS now faces. In brief, they can contribute to improved performance, however they most likely cannot become new 'magic bullets' which alone could transform the NHS sufficiently to guarantee its future.

The role of predictive technologies in healthcare

Marco Viceconti

The practice of medicine is largely an exercise in prediction. A patient goes to see the doctor, who collects a series of observations about the patient and uses them to predict the underlying cause of the symptoms (diagnosis), the severity of the possibly outcomes (prognosis), or the appropriateness of different interventions (treatment planning). It is all about predicting, from what we know about the patient and from the vast body of specialist knowledge we can access, some other things we do not know about the patient, but that we need to know in order to take the medical decision.

So why for many authors is the future of healthcare, to use the words of Auffray, Charron, and Hood,[1] a 'Predictive, personalised, preventive, and participative' medicine? Didn't we just say that the practice of medicine is mostly about predicting?

Traditionally prediction in medicine is done by homology.[2] Based on past experience, we know that if the patient exhibits certain signs we can assume that in some regards he/she is akin to a group of past patients who showed the same signs and where treated in a certain way got better. But of course things are never so simple. No two patients are identical (studies on the most similar humans, monozygotic twins, show how differently they develop diseases[3][4][5][6][7][8] so our patients will exhibit clearly only some of the signs that characterised that group of past patients. As a result these reference groups, produced in controlled clinical studies that provide the evidences on which most medical decisions are based, tend to be formed by very many persons, who are equal only in regard of a very few signs, many less of all those that may influence the appearance, the severity, or the response to treatment of a certain disease. In other words, medicine is not very personalised.

A new generation of healthcare technologies, largely still under development, promise to charge this scenario quite radically. They make it possible to collect a large amount of clinically relevant signs of each patient in a quantitative way, with excellent accuracy, and progressively lower costs; they allow this large volume of information on each patient to be handled entirely in digital format, and to be managed efficiently so that the medical professional can have all information when necessary, where necessary, and presented in the most significant way; and most important these technologies can generate patient-specific computer simulations that can support the medical decision in a much more accurate and personalised way. We call these predictive medicine technologies.[9][10][11][12][13]

There is a fundamental difference between the predictions a doctor makes based on evidences and those these patient-specific models provide. As we explained the earlier are done by homology; the latter are done by analogy.[14] The patient-specific model in the computer is not the patient; it does not even resemble the patient. But the evolution of the disease over time, or the effect of a treatment on that patient that the model predicts, is analogous to what we will eventually observe on the real patient. This analogy is established by capturing into the model the vast amount of knowledge we have on how the human body works from a physical, chemical, physiological and biological point of view; with this knowledge, if we provide the model with a lot of quantitative data on how things are in that patient now, it will be able to predict quite accurately how things will become in the future, under certain circumstances.

We should not fall into the 'avatar' trap, and evoke the image of a virtual replica of the patient, with all its characteristics: a patient-specific model does not and cannot predict everything that happens in the patient body; each model is designed to predict a very specific manifestation of the patient body, which we know to be essential to take the most appropriate medical decision. One of the earliest predictive medicine technologies made available for general clinical use predicts how the blood flows in a small network of blood vessels that wrap the heart, and how it would flow after we dilate by a few millimetres a small section of one of these vessels that a disease has narrowed; the question might seem trivial, but the answer is incredibly complicated, and only 10 years ago it would have been impossible to answer accurately.[15][16]

In cases like this clinicians take a decision mostly as an educated guess, supplementing the few evidences available with their professional experience; but it is not unusual that after a complex and expensive intervention the patient shows no significant benefit, and further interventions are required. Predictive medicine technologies promise better-informed medical decisions, with significant improvement of the efficacy of care. The ability to accurately predict enables a much more personalised medicine, where the prediction, and thus the decision based upon it, takes into account many more factors specific to the patient than we can possibly do today. The area where this is particularly critical is prevention: only with a predictive medicine capable of a much higher level of personalisation we will be able to recognise those who are at risk, and the best way to prevent that risk becoming a reality.

Last, but definitely not least, we believe predictive medicine can enable a much more participative medicine. The role that the patient should play in the medical decision process is a very complex topic, in which technologies probably play a marginal role. But if a technology makes it possible for the medical professional to describe to the patient, with a much higher level of confidence than today is possible, what is the most likely outcome for each of the available treatment options, a more participative medicine becomes a much more realistic objective. An example: cancer in elder patients poses frequently a risk of therapeutic obstinacy; but the decision to choose a palliative therapy that improves the quality of the remaining life as opposed to a much more aggressive therapy aimed to extend life expectancy is difficult to choose when there is a large uncertainty of how the patient will respond to that more aggressive therapy.

What does all this have to do with the future of universal healthcare? This technology promise to drastically improve the accuracy of many critical decisions, improving the outcome and ensuring we spend money in expensive therapies where we know they will work. It allows to account better for individual differences, and to consider complex determinants such as lifestyle, which again can only improve the cost-effectiveness of healthcare spending. It makes prevention, early diagnosis, and early treatment a much more likely reality, thanks to our improved ability to predict what will happen in a year, in five years, in 10 years in regard to a specific medical question. And by increasing the ability of the medical professionals to know in advance the effect of each available choice, it makes much more real the concept of patient participation.

In the following pages we will explain what predictive medicine technologies can currently do through some selected examples, what the most advanced research projects promise it can achieve in a few years, and which type of healthcare model could emerge once these technologies are fully developed and adopted. Last we will briefly discuss the role that technological innovation in general could play in our hospitals.

Predictive medicine today

New predictive medicine technologies are proposed in the specialised literature every day, so providing an exhaustive overview of what is available in the research labs worldwide is beyond the scope of this chapter. Here we will describe a few selected examples, chosen because they are closer to the full clinical adoption, or because they address conditions of particular socioeconomic importance.[17]

In the author's knowledge the first predictive medicine technology to achieve approval from the USA Food and Drug Administration belongs to a special group where the quantity to be predicted can indeed be measured directly, but through a costly, invasive and/or dangerous procedure. Fractional flow reserve (FFR) expresses the pressure drop across a narrowing (stenosis) of one of the blood vessels that wrap the heart (coronaries); it can be measured by inserting through an endovascular procedure an instrumented catheter across the stenosis. While it has been proved that FFR has an accuracy of more than 90% in identifying if the stenosis is causing cardiac ischemia,[18] this procedure is rarely used because of the cost, complexity, and risk that the direct measurement of the FFR involves. Using a patient-specific model generated from coronary computed tomographic angiography images, the HeartFlow service[19] can predict non invasively the value of the FFR.[20] The HeartFlow technology received full FDA approval recently, and is now available for use worldwide. In the UK, the Insigneo institute in Sheffield has completed a phase one clinical trial on a similar solution that uses rotational coronary angiography, which is far more accessible than CT angiography, especially in Europe.[21]

A similar application also developed by Insigneo, which has just completed the phase one trial, makes it possible to perform an accurate differential diagnosis of pulmonary hypertension without the need for a delicate invasive right heart catheterisation, the current standard of care.[22]

Complex cardiac surgeries, such as transcatheter aortic valve implantation (TAVI), or paediatric percutaneous pulmonary valve implantation, require accurate planning in order to be successful. A new generation of predictive medicine technologies allow performing a patient-specific simulation of the device deployment, and to predict how it will perform if deployed in that way in that patient. An excellent work was done recently on a particularly difficult paediatric case at the Great Ormond Street Hospital for Children in London.[23] A Dutch start-up, FEOPS,[24] is testing a software technology called TAVIGuide, to assist with the planning of TAVI procedures.

Aneurysms are localised bulges that form in the wall of a blood vessel. In many cases we can live all our lives with an aneurysm without even knowing it, as they are frequently totally asymptomatic. But if the aneurysm is detected, the clinical specialist must decide whether to treat it, which usually involves some serious risks, or leave it alone with the risk that the lesion keeps growing and eventually bursts, producing a massive haemorrhage. So predicting the risk of rupture of individual aneurysms remains one of the holy grails for predictive medicine research. But the problem is incredibly complex, and all technologies are in the early stages of development. Some interesting results were obtained for abdominal aortic aneurysms,[25] while for cerebral aneurysms a lot more research is required.

For the musculoskeletal system one of the first clinical problems tackled by predictive medicine technologies was the risk of bone fracture in osteoporotic patients.[27] [28] [29] [30] [31] Today, the Insigneo predictive technology can correctly discriminate in retrospective studies fractured and non-fractured patients with an accuracy of 75%-84%, depending on the age distribution of the patients.

Whole body musculoskeletal patient-specific models are also used in the treatment planning of paediatric cerebral palsy patients.[32] [33] [34] [35] [36] [37] [38] [39] Another interesting target is oncology, for example, predicting the response for individual patients with breast cancer undergoing neo-adjuvant therapy.[40]

Predictive medicine tomorrow

From the few examples provided in the previous section it is easy to notice that the low-hanging fruits for predictive medicine are those conditions where the quantity to be predicted is related to a physical event, such as rupture, fracture, flow resistance, etc. These events are particularly important for the cardiovascular-respiratory, and the neuromusculoskeletal systems and their pathologies. Thus, it is easy to forecast the first wave of predictive medicine technologies that will hit the clinics in the next five years will target these conditions. For specific pathologies/interventions the specialist will take his/her decision supported by the predictions of a patient-specific model. This should improve the success rate of these procedures, reduce the complications, but more important for the topic at hand increase the appropriateness of these complex and very expensive interventions, that will be performed only where a concrete benefit is predicted for that patient, avoiding unnecessary discomfort for the patient and unnecessary costs for the healthcare system.

Oncology requires more complex models, where the physical interaction of the tumour mass that is growing with the surrounding tissues, but also the metabolism of the various cellular populations in relation to their mutations, the degree of vascularisation, the tumour mass heterogeneity, etc. Still, the recent work by Weis *et al.* suggests, at least for breast cancer, an accuracy of 87% in predicting how the tumour mass changes in each patient as a function of the treatment.[41] In these models we are building an essential bridge between the physiology-based models that describe processes as the tissue organ and organism scales, and the system biology models that mostly describe processes within a single cell, at the molecular scale. Once this very challenging connection is completed the ability of predictive medicine technologies to deliver will be extended to all those conditions where the disease and its treatment are the result of complex interactions between genetic and epigenetic determinants.

In general this first wave of technologies will have the medical professional as end user, to whom they will provide decision support, providing a much more personalised medicine, an increase in appropriateness, and hopefully also a reduction in adverse effects, complications, and medical errors. A second wave, whose development is starting only now on a large scale, are the so-called in silico clinical trial technologies. Early examples are the Cobelli-Kovatchev diabetes simulator,[42] which the FDA has approved as a replacement to animal experimentation in the pre-clinical assessment of new artificial pancreas technologies, or the Virtual Assay software developed by the team of Blanca Rodriguez at the University of Oxford, which can screen new compounds for the risk of cardiotoxicity.[43] In both cases, the predictive medicine technologies are used to reduce, refine, or partially replace animal experimentation. But we start to see examples where such technologies are also used to augment clinical trials in humans,[44] making it possible to investigate the safety and efficacy of a new drug or medical device in a range of conditions much wider than any traditional clinical trial could allow. Here the expected long-term advantage is to reduce the costs of innovation in healthcare, reduce the time to market, while at the same time improve the safety of the new biomedical products being tested.[45]

The last, longer-term application, is referred in some documents are personal health forecasting. The idea is to combine predictive medicine technologies that run in real time or quasi-real time with mobile health technologies as wearable sensors, so that as physiological signals, lifestyle determinants, or other patient-provided information are collected, a predictive medicine model is run and a prediction is updated, to be returned to the patient for information, support to self-management, and strengthen behavioural change applications. It is easy to see how such technologies would be game-changers for preventive medicine, and for the management outside the hospital of chronic, age-related conditions.

Predictive medicine based universal healthcare

So let's assume that some time in the future all these research activities will be successfully completed, and predictive medicine will become a fully accomplished reality. Which model of healthcare provision would it enable?

The most visible difference would be the role that information technology plays in the healthcare industry. Wearable sensors will continuously monitor our physiological signals and store them safely in the cloud, where the patient can retrieve them at any time, or grant access to them to any medical professional. If the patient agrees to become a 'data donor' all these digital data are also copied (in anonymised form) together with those of thousands of other citizens in immense data warehouses, where they are continuously analysed by automated programs that seek interesting patterns and correlations. Last, this healthcare cloud would allow searching anonymously for all people whose health data match a certain health pattern, and send them lifestyle recommendations, invitations to tests, and in general anything that can help prevention.

When a subject is found to be at risk for a particular disease, he/she would be asked to wear extra sensors that collect more specific information related to that condition, and his/her data are linked to a specific personal health forecasting service; all physiological data collected daily would then be processed in real time by this patient-specific model, which would return personalised suggestions, produce evidences that can be used for behavioural changes, and where necessary raise alarms to the GP.

GP consultations would involve access to all available data; to keep the duration of these visits down, very advanced big data exploration software should be available, so that the GP can quickly navigate this deluge of data and find the specific set of information required. Pharmacies would become much more points of care, where prescriptions are collected, and additional examinations that can be highly automated are performed, so as to avoid overloading GP surgeries or hospitals for things such as a blood test. But everything would be automatically stored in the citizen health cloud, and retrieved by anyone authorised, anywhere, at anytime.

But medical professionals would rarely access the raw data. Most of the time they would base their decision on predictive medicine technologies that would 'digest' large amounts of data on the subject and provide the predictions required to support that particular decision. User interfaces will probably evolve to provide a very interactive environment, possibly with vocal interfaces like Apple SIRI,[46] so that the doctor explores the available information in any way he/she likes, rather than being forced into a rigid pre-defined process.

A&E will be particularly transformed by these technologies. First, prevention will drastically reduce the number of citizens who access A&E services; also, the flexibility of digital technologies will allow them to handle many situations during nights and weekends at home, as the remote medical professional can talk to the patient face to face with telemedicine technologies, and with the patient permission query all his/her health data. A nurse could be sent to the home of the patient, and instructed remotely by the specialists. Overall the emergency response should be able to grade the response much better and use hospital accesses only as an extreme ratio. Also emergency admissions would be radically transformed if the patient arrives 'escorted' by the totality of his/her health data for emergency A&E specialists to access.

The ability to monitor almost continuously the vital signs of a patient anywhere, and for predictive medicine technologies to process a large volume of data into useful facts to support the medical decision, would expand immensely the scope of day hospital organisational models. Large hospitals hosting all medical specialisms would manage over the territory a network of smaller clinics where patients are admitted for a few hours or a night at most and receive procedures from non-specialised medical professionals guided by remote specialists, who can monitor in real time all vital signs.

A common procedure in these day hospitals would be to deploy ingestible, injectable or implantable sensors designed to monitor for a short amount of time much more detailed signals. The patient would be admitted to the day hospital, receive a specific sensor, and then discharged while his vital signs are closely monitored and analysed while the patient goes about with his/her normal life. A few days later he/she could go back to have the sensor removed, and the optimal treatment – selected by the specialist based on the prediction of a patient-specific model – is performed.

The common element of this narrative is that information is plentiful and accessible anywhere, and predictive medicine technologies let the citizen, his carers, or the medical professionals who are serving him/her to obtain quickly, precisely and clearly the information required to take the most appropriate decision. Healthcare infrastructures become much cheaper, lightweight and flexible, with the logic that data rather than people move around.

Technological innovation: a core business for the hospitals of the future

How credible is the scenario above, in the light of the incredible slow rate of adoption of technologies in healthcare? How can we imagine such a broad information management vision when most hospitals today struggle in managing just the small amount of information produced within their walls?

Universal healthcare providers such as the NHS are mostly organisations oriented to the provision of service. As such they tend to focus on the reliability of the services they provide, rather than their ability to change.

The tremendous budgetary pressure that NHS organisations have been exposed to in the last years has made this process even worse: most hospitals today focus on being able to continue providing a similar quality of services while staffing is being reduced, instrumentations become obsolete, and infrastructures are not properly maintained. In all this there is little time and patience for innovation.

But in our opinion the problem runs deeper. Some years ago, when in many European countries the cost of universal healthcare started to be become unbearable, outsourcing became a popular strategy. Mimicking other industrial sectors, hospitals started to buy from external companies those services that – while contributing considerably to the operational costs – were perceived not to be part of the 'core business' of the organisation. The first services to be outsourced were catering and cleaning, but in many hospitals also information technology services were outsourced,[47] sometimes with disastrous results. How could some healthcare organisations decide that IT services were not core business, when a hospital is first and foremost an organisation that produces and manages information?

Historically medicine and biology are somehow perceived alternatives to mathematics and engineering in our educational systems. If you are gifted with numbers you will be an engineer, if you are not, you will be a doctor. So historically doctors received very little education around technology, and they have little understanding of it. While a modern hospital sees the contribution of many professions, the top management of almost every hospital has mostly a biomedical background. It is quite normal to consider not so important what we do not fully understand, so it should not come as a surprise if technological innovation has not been at the core of healthcare organisations in UK.

Technological innovation in healthcare is something that nowadays happens mostly outside our hospitals. A company decides there is a need, usually on the basis of marketing considerations, develops a technology targeting what is usually considered a high-risk, high-margin, low volumes market, makes a significant investment in R&D and to pass the EC mark check for safety, and then starts to push the technology onto the healthcare market. In countries lucky enough to have an organisation like NICE, someone tries hard to see if the increase of cost that the technology involves brings a proportionate benefit, and if this seems the case the new technology starts to be reimbursed by the universal healthcare system. In countries like the USA where the customer is the patient it is enough to show that some benefit exists, no matter what the cost is. As a result most analysts agree that adding technology usually increases the costs. But this is in stark opposition to almost any other industrial sector where technology nearly always reduces costs.

We propose that the root of the problem is who drives the technological development. If we can bring technological innovation at the core of each hospital, new technologies will emerge that are designed to target the need of universal healthcare provision, and not of the health technology market. Most of these technologies will be based on consumer electronics and open-source software, with drastically lower costs. Hospitals will handle the de-risking and certification process directly, confirm the cost-benefit ratio for each new technology, and then contract external companies to manufacture them in volume under license. These same companies could also commercialise NHS-owned innovations in other countries, again under some licensing contracts. Alternatively, hospitals could spin off companies that produce, commercialise, and provide deployment and training services on a selected piece of technology developed by that hospital to other hospitals in this and other countries.

A last point is related to the total cost of care. Most disruptive technologies, including predictive medicine ones, tend to change the clinical pathway (and this is sometimes the biggest benefit to harvest). Because of this, the cost-benefit analyses are usually difficult to conduct. If we look at the clinical pathway augmented by predictive technologies we may find that the total cost in imaging has increased, and new extra costs of processing and computing appear that were not present in the previous pathway. Based on these partial analyses it is easy to conclude that these technologies are not cost-effective. But to reach a solid conclusion one has to look at the total cost of care, which includes not only the secondary care costs, but also the primary ones, and if possible also the social costs (work loss, time of family carers, etc.) A global provider like the NHS should in theory be in the best position to promote any means that reduce the total cost of care for a disease, regardless of how these costs are moved around within the healthcare system.

Notes

A public health perspective
John Ashton

1   Sir W. Beveridge, 'Social Insurance and Allied Services', Cmd, 6404, 6405, HMSO, London, 1942.

2   NHS England, 'Five Year Forward View', London, NHS England, 2014.

3   World Health Organisation, 'Declaration of Alma Ata', Geneva, WHO, UNICEF, 1978.

4   World Health Organisation, 'Global Strategy for Health For All by the Year 2000', Geneva, WHO, 1981.

5   J. Ashton and H. Seymour, *The New Public Health*, Milton Keynes, Open University Press, 1988.

6   H. Vuori,'Primary Health Care in Industrialised Countries', *Die Allgemeinpraxix; Das Zentrum Der Artzlichen, Grundverorgung Gottlieb Duttwierer*, Zurich, InstitutRuschlikon, 1981, pp. 83-111.

7   'Community Control of Cardiovascular Diseases, The North Karelia Project', Published on behalf of the National Public Health Laboratory of Finland by the WHO Regional Office for Europe, 1981.

8   A. Oakley and J. Barker (eds), *Private Complaints and Public Health: Richard Titmusson the National Health Service*, Bristol, The Policy Press, 2004.

9   P. Townsend and N. Davidson, *Inequalities in Health – The Black Report*, Harmondsworth, Penguin, 1980.

10 M. Marmot, *The Health Gap: The Challenge of an Unequal World*, London, Bloomsbury, 2015.

11 S. Monaghan, D. Huws and M. Navarro, 'The Case for a New UK Health for the People Act', London, The Nuffield Trust, 2003.

12 I. Illich, *Medical Nemesis – The Expropriation of Health*, London, Marion Boyars, 1975.

13 J. McKnight, *The Careless Society*, New York, Perseus Books, 1995.

14 L. Levin, A. Katz, and E. Holst, *Self-Care*, London, Vroom Helm, 1977.

15 L. S. Levin and E. C. Idler, *The Hidden Health Care System – Social Resources in Health Care*, Golden Apple Publications, 2010.

16 J. McKnight and P. Block, *The Abundant Community, Awakening the Power of Families and Neighbourhoods*, American Planning Association, San Francisco, California, Berrett-Koehler Publishers, 2010.

17 R. D. Putnam, *Bowling Alone*, New York, Simon Schuster, 2000.

18 With acknowledgements to Chris Gates.

19 S. L. Kark, *The Practice of Community Orientated Primary Care*, New York, Appleton-Century-Crofts, 1981.

20 J. Ashton, P. Grey and K. Barnard, 'Healthy Cities – WHO's New Public Health Initiative', *Health Promotion*, vol. 1, no. 3, 1986, pp. 319-324.

21 G. Caplan, *An Approach to Community Mental Health*, London, Tavistock Publications, 1961.

22 C. Winslow, The Untilled Fields of Public Health, *Science*, vol. 51, no. 1306, 1920, pp. 23-33.

Postcards from the frontline

Melanie Reid

1 'Cancelled Elective Operations Data', NHS England, 2015, https://www.england.nhs.uk/statistics/statistical-work-areas/cancelled-elective-operations/cancelled-ops-data/.

2 B. Irvine, 'Social insurance the right way forward for health care in the United Kingdom? For Against', *BMJ*, vol. 325 no. 488, 2002, http://www.bmj.com/content/325/7362/488

3 D. Green, B. Irvine E. Clarke, E. Bidgood, 'Health Systems: France', Civitas, 2013, http://www.civitas.org.uk/nhs/download/france.pdf

4 D. Green, B. Irvine, E. Clarke, E. Bidgood, 'Health Systems: France', Civitas, 2013 http://www.civitas.org.uk/nhs/download/france.pdf

5 D. Green, B. Irvine, E. Clarke, E. Bidgood, 'Health Systems: France', Civitas, 2013 http://www.civitas.org.uk/nhs/download/france.pdf

6 'Future trends', The King's Fund, 2015 http://www.kingsfund.org.uk/time-to-think-differently/trends

7 T. Fleming, M. Robinson, B. Thomson, N. Graetz, C. Margono, E. Mullany, S. Biryukov, C. Abbafati, , S. Abera, J. Abraham, N. Abu-Rmeileh, T. Achoki, F. AlBuhairan, Z. Alemu, *et al.*, 'Global, regional, and national prevalence of overweight and obesity in

children and adults during 1980-2013: a systematic analysis for the Global Burden of Disease Study 2013', *The Lancet*, vol. 384, 2014, pp 766-781.

8   'Diabetes Prevalence 2014', Diabetes UK, 2014 https://www.diabetes.org.uk/About_us/What-we-say/Statistics/Diabetes-prevalence-2014/

9   '2015 Manifesto: Eight practical recommendations to prevent obesity and type 2 diabetes', Action on Sugar, 2014 http://www.actiononsalt.org.uk/actiononsugar/Press%20Release%20/141202.pdf

10 'Foresight: Tackling Obesities, Future Choices Project Report', Government Office for Science, 2007 https://www.gov.uk/government/uploads/system/uploads/attachment_data/file/287937/07-1184x-tackling-obesities-future-choices-report.pdf

11 N. Hex, C. Barlett, D. Wight, M. Taylor, D. Varley, 'Estimating the current and future costs of Type 1 and Type 2 diabetes in the UK, including direct health costs and indirect societal and productivity costs', *Diabet Med*, vol. 29, no. 7, 2012,1 pp855-62.

12 '2015 Manifesto: Eight practical recommendations to prevent obesity and type 2 diabetes', Action on Sugar, 2014, http://www.actiononsalt.org.uk/actiononsugar/Press%20Release%20/141202.pdf

13 J. Horton, 'Private care centres 'will aid NHS', *The Sunday Times*, 2015, http://www.thesundaytimes.co.uk/sto/news/uk_news/scotland/article1594402.ece

14 D. Green, B. Irvine, E. Clarke, E. Bidgood, 'Health Systems: Germany', Civitas, 2013 http://www.civitas.org.uk/nhs/download/germany.pdf

15 A. Fahy, F. Wong, K. Kunasingam, D. Neen, F. Dockery, A. Ajuied, D. Back, 'A Review of Hip Fracture Mortality—Why and How Does Such a Large Proportion of These Elderly Patients Die?' *Sugical Science*, vol. 5, 2014, pp.227-232, http://www.scirp.org/journal/PaperInformation.aspx?PaperID=46295

16 'Data Briefing: Emergency bed use: what the numbers tell us', The King's Fund, 2011, http://www.kingsfund.org.uk/sites/files/kf/data-briefing-emergency-bed-use-what-the-numbers-tell-us-emmi-poteliakhoff-james-thompson-kings-fund-december-2011.pdf

17 'Protecting fragile bones: A strategy to reduce the impact of osteoporosis and fragility in fractures in Wales', National Osteoporosis Society, 2009, https://www.nos.org.uk/NetCommunity/Document.Doc?id=491

18 'Call to Action: Hip fractures are breaking the bank and lives -
    Are you ready to stop the UK reaching 'Breaking Point'?'
    International Longevity Society, 2010, http://www.thebms.org.uk/
    publicdownloads/Call_to_Action_Politicians.PDF

19 J. Tusa, 'The BBC and the licence fee revolution', *The Times*, 2015
    http://www.thetimes.co.uk/tto/opinion/letters/article450130
    6.ece

20 'Softly does it', The Economist, 2015, http://www.
    economist.com/news/britain/21657655-oxbridge-one-direction-
    and-premier-league-bolster-britains-power-persuade-softly-
    does-it

21 'NHS payout of £50,000 for nurse', Herand Scotland, 2012
    http://www.heraldscotland.com/news/13082003.NHS_payout
    _of___50_000_for_nurse/

22 R. Feneley, C. Kunin, D. Stickler, 'An indwelling urinary catheter
    for the 21st century', *BJU Int*, vol. 109, no. 12, 2011, pp 1746-9,
    http://www.ncbi.nlm.nih.gov/pubmed/22094023

23 'Urinary Tract Infection (Catheter-Associated Urinary Tract
    Infection [CAUTI] and Non-Catheter-Associated Urinary Tract
    Infection [UTI]) and Other Urinary System Infection [USI]) Events',
    CDC, 2016 http://www.cdc.gov/nhsn/PDFs/pscManual/
    7pscCAUTIcurrent.pdf

24 R. Feneley, 'Innovation, Health and Wealth', NHS Instiute
    for Innovation and Improvement, 2011, http://
    www.institute.nhs.uk/images//documents/Innovation/Innov
    ation%20Health%20and%20Wealth%20-%20accelerating%
    20adoption%20and%20diffusion%20in%20the%20NHS.pdf

25 A. Chapple, S. Prinjha, R. Feneley, S. Zebland, 'Drawing
    on Accounts of Long-Term Urinary Catheter Use: Design for
    the Seemingly Mundane', *Quality Health Res*, 2015, pii:
    1049732315570135,
    http://www.ncbi.nlm.nih.gov/pubmed/25646001

26 A. Roberts, V. Wells, L. Czaplewski, 'Living in a world without
    anitbioltics', Proceedings of the British Science Festival,
    University of Bradford, 2015, https://www.biochemistry.org/
    Events/tabid/379/MeetingNo/P_P_PE_BSAfestival/view/Co
    nference/Default.aspx

A health service (re)designed to help doctors give the best possible care to their patients

Mark Porter and Sally Al-Zaidy

1   British Medical Association, *Proposals for a General Medical Service for the Nation*, London: BMA, 1930.

2   British Medical Association, *A General Medical Service for the Nation*, London: BMA, 1938.

3   British Medical Association, *Public health and healthcare delivery task and finish group final report*. London BMA, 2015.

4   L. A. Aday, R. M. Andersen, 'Equity of Access to Medical Care: a conceptual and empirical overview', Medical Care, vol. XIX, no. 12, 1981.

5   M. Koivusalo, K. Wyss, P. Santana, Chapter 11 'Effects of decentralisation and recentralisation on equity dimensions of health systems', Saltman R B, Bankauskaite V, Vrangbæk K (eds.) *Decentralisation in Health Care*, McGraw-Hill Open University Press, 2007.

6   S. Al-Zaidy, *Concepts of equity in the NHS: What do doctors understand by universality and comprehensiveness?* London: BMA, 2013.

7   A. Wagstaff, E. van Doorslaer, H. van der Burg et al., 'Equity in the Finance of Health Care: Some Further International Comparisons', *Journal of Health Economics*, vol.18, 1999, pp. 263-90.

8   C. LaMontagne, *NerdWallet Health Study: Medical debt crisis worsening despite health care policy advances*, NerdWallet, 2014, http://www.nerdwallet.com/blog/health/2014/10/08/medical-bills-debt-crisis/

9   Op. cit. *Public health and healthcare delivery task and finish group final report.*

10 H. Hogan, R. Zipfel, J. Neuburger, A. Hutchings, A. Darzi, N. Black, 'Availability of hospital deaths and association with hospital-wide mortality ratios: retrospective case record review and regression analysis', *BMJ*, vol. 351, h3239, 2015.

11 R. Klein, J. Maybin, *Thinking about rationing*, London: King's Fund, 2012.

12 *Ibid.*

13 S. Al-Zaidy, *National versus local equity: How much variation is acceptable to doctors?*, London: BMA, 2013.

14 *Value based clinical commissioning of elective surgical care*, RightCare, 2011.

15 *Setting priorities in health: the challenge for clinical commissioning. Research summary*, London: Nuffield Trust, 2012.

16 S. Al-Zaidy, *Balancing the books: What types of rationing are most acceptable to doctors?*, London: BMA, 2013.

17 S. Clark, A. Weale, 'Social values in health priority setting: a conceptual framework', *Journal of Health Organization and Management*, vol. 26, no. 3, 2012.

18 Op. cit. *Balancing the books: What types of rationing are most acceptable to doctors?*

19 *The NHS Atlas of Variation in Healthcare: reducing unwarranted variation to increase value and improve quality.* RightCare, London: Public Health England, 2015.

20 *Value based clinical commissioning of elective surgical care,* RightCare, 2011.

21 *Ibid.*

22 Op. cit. *Thinking about rationing.*

23 *BMJ Clinical Evidence Handbook,* London: BMJ Group, BMJ, 2011.

24 *NICE 'do not do' recommendations* https://www.nice.org.uk/news/article/cut-nhs-waste-through-nice%E2%80%99s-%E2%80%98do-not-do%E2%80%99-database

25 *Five year forward view: time to delivery,* London: NHS England, 2015.

26 *The five year forward view,* London: NHS England, 2014.

27 Op. cit. *A General Medical Service for the Nation.*

28 Op. cit. *Public health and healthcare delivery task and finish group final report.*

29 *Ibid.*

30 Canadian Institute of Advanced Research, Health Canada, Population and Public Health Branch, AB/NWT 2002, quoted in D. Kuznetsova, 2012, *Healthy places: Councils leading on public health,* London: New Local Government Network. http://www.nlgn.org.uk/public/wp-content/uploads/Healthy-Places_FINAL.pdf

31 *Health inequalities widen within most areas of England,* UCL Institute of Health Equity press release, 2012.

32 *Health policy under the coalition government.* London: The Kings Fund, 2012.

33 *Growing up in the UK: ensuring a healthy future for our children,* British Medical Association, London: BMA, 2013.

34 *Prioritising health and wellbeing in social and economic policy,* British Medical Association (unpublished), London: BMA.

35 *Marmot indicators 2014.* A preliminary summary with graphs, London: Institute of Health Equity, 2014.

36 *Public sector employment, Q2, September 2014,* Newport: Office for National Statistics, 2014.

37 K. Leppo. E. Ollila, S. Pena, M, Wismar. S. Cook, *Health in all policies: seizing opportunities, implementing policies,* Finland: Ministry of Social Affairs and Health, 2013.

38   L. Brereton, V. Vasoodaven, 'The impact of the NHS market: an overview of the literature', Civitas, 2010.

39   *Competition in the NHS*, London: Office of Health Economics, 2012.

40   C. Paton, *At what cost? Paying the price for the market in the English NHS*. Centre for Health and the Public Interest, 2014.

41   M. Fotaki, *What market-based choice can't do for the NHS: the theory and evidence of how choice works in healthcare*, Centre for Health and the Public Interest, 2014.

42   Op. cit. *At what cost? Paying the price for the market in the English NHS.*

43   N. Timmins, 'The four UK health systems Learning from each other', London: The King's Fund, 2013.

44   Op. cit. *Public health and healthcare delivery task and finish group final report*

45   *Annual Report and Accounts 2014-15*, London: Department of Health, 2015.

46   *Western Sussex Hospitals NHS Foundation Trust and NHS Coastal West Sussex Clinical Commissioning Group: Summary of the review of financial, clinical and operational impact of the MSK service tender*, PricewaterhouseCoopers, 2014.

47   C. Clough, *Final report: Independent review of Nottingham dermatology services*. NHS Rushcliffe Clinical Commissioning Group, 2015.

On the brink of disruption: how can universal healthcare make the most of radical innovation?

Steve Melton

1   C. Deutsch, 'At Kodak, Some Old Things Are New Again', *The New York Times*, 2008, http://www.nytimes.com/2008/05/02/technology/02kodak.html?_r=0

2   'Sales of Digital Cameras Decline as Consumers Snap Up Smartphones', Mintel, 2012, http://www.mintel.com/press-centre/technology-press-centre/sales-of-digital-cameras-decline-as-consumers-snap-up-smartphones

3   'The number of hospital beds', The King's Fund, 2015, http://www.kingsfund.org.uk/projects/nhs-in-a-nutshell/hospital-beds

4   D. Whitehouse, 'Tattoos to 3D printing: five inventions that will revolutionaise healthcare', *The Guardian*, 2015, http://www.theguardian.com/healthcare-network/2015/sep/04/tattoos-to-3d-printing-five-inventions-that-will-revolutionise-healthcare

5   'Key Stats', Age UK London, 2015, http://www.ageuk.org.uk/
    london/about-age-uk-london/media-centre/key-stats/

6   'How does health spending in the United Kingdom compare?',
    OECD, 2015 http://www.oecd.org/unitedkingdom/Country-
    Note-UNITED%20KINGDOM-OECD-Health-Statistics-2015.pdf

7   J. Boucher, 'The Nobel Prize: Excellence among Immigrants',
    George Mason Institute for Immigration, 2013 http://
    s3.amazonaws.com/chssweb/documents/20864/original/Nob
    el_Prize_Research_Brief_Final.pdf?1447975594

Turning healthcare on its head: the bidet revolution

Phil Hammond

1   E. Crawley, A. Emond, J. Sterne, 'Unidentified Chronic Fatigue
    Syndrome/myalgic encephalomyelitis (CFS/ME) is a major
    cause of school absence: surveillance outcomes from school-
    based clinics', *BMJ Open*, vol. 1, no. 2, :e000252, 2011.

2   E. Crawley, 'The epidemiology of chronic fatigue syndrome/
    myalgic encephalitis in children', *Arch Dis Child*, 2013.

3   E, Crawley, J. Sterne, 'Association between school absence and
    physical function in paediatric chronic fatigue syndrome/
    myalgic encephalopathy', *Arch Dis Child*, vol. 94, no. 10, 2009,
    pp. 752-56.

4   L. Rangel, M. Garralda, M. Levin *et al.*,'The course of severe
    chronic fatigue syndrome in childhood' *JRSocMed*, vol. 93, no.3,
    2000, pp. 129-34.

5   A. Missen, W. Hollingworth, N. Eaton, *et al.*, 'The financial and
    psychological impacts on mothers of children with chronic
    fatigue syndrome (CFS/ME)', *Child Care Health Dev*, vol.38, no.4,
    2012, pp. 505-12.

6   C. Webb, S. Collin, T. Deave *et al.*, 'What stops children with
    a chronic illness accessing health care: a mixed methods
    study in children with Chronic Fatigue Syndrome/Myalgic
    Encephalomyelitis (CFS/ME)', *BMC Health Serv Res*, vol. 11 no.
    1, 2011, p. 308.

7   S. Nijhof, G. Bleijenberg, C. Uiterwaal *et al.*, 'Effectiveness of
    internet-based cognitive behavioural treatment for adolescents
    with chronic fatigue syndrome (FITNET): a randomised
    controlled trial', *Lancet*; vol. 379, no. 9824, 2012, pp. 1412-8.

Three challenges for the future: funding, integration and the workforce

Richard Murray

1   Ipsos MORI, *Trust in professions*, 5 Jan 2015. Available at: Ipsos MORI (accessed on 25 September 2015). https://www.ipsos-mori.com/researchpublications/researcharchive/15/Trust-in-Profressions.aspx

2   The Commonwealth Fund, *International Profiles of Health Care Systems, 2014: Australia, Canada, Denmark, England, France, Germany, Italy, Japan, The Netherlands, New Zealand, Norway, Singapore, Sweden, Switzerland, and the United States*, New York, The Commonwealth Fund, 2015, (accessed 25 September 2015).

3   Appleby, J and R. Robertson, *British Social Attitudes 2014. Public satisfaction with the NHS and healthcare*, London, The King's Fund, 2015.

4   NHS England, Care Quality Commission, Health Education England, Monitor, Public Health England, NHS Trust Development Authority, *NHS five year forward view*, London, NHS England, 2014.

5   OECD, *Health at a Glance 2013: OECD indicators*, OECD Publishing, Paris, 2013.

6   The King's Fund, *Spending Review submission: health and social care funding*, London, The King's Fund, 2015b.

7   The King's Fund, *Quarterly Monitoring Report July 2015: how is the NHS performing?* London, The King's Fund, 2015a. Available at: The King's Fund (accessed 25 September 2015).

8   Association of Greater Manchester Authorities, NHS England, Greater Manchester Association of Clinical Commissioning Groups, *Greater Manchester Health and Social Care Devolution. Memorandum of Understanding*, Manchester, Association of Greater Manchester Authorities, 2015. Available from: Association of Greater Manchester Authorities (accessed 25 September 2015)

9   Commission on the Future of Health and Social Care in England, *A new settlement for health and social care*, London, The King's Fund, 2014.

10 Buck, D. and D. Maguire, *Inequalities in life expectancy.* Changes over time and implications for policy, London, The King's Fund, 2015.

11 The King's Fund and the Local Government Association, *Making the case for public health interventions*, London, The King's Fund, 2014. Available at: The King's Fund (accessed 25 September 2015).

12   Department of Health, *The NHS Plan: a plan for investment, a plan for reform*, Command Paper 4818-I, 2000.

13   Addicott, R., Maguire, D., Honeyman, M., and J.Jabbal, *Workforce Planning in the NHS*, London, The King's Fund, 2015.

14   The Royal College of General Practitioners and the Royal Pharmaceutical Society, *RCGP and RPS Policy Statement on GP practice based pharmacists*, RCGP/RPS, 2015. Available at: RPS (accessed 25 September 2015).

15   Addicott, R., Maguire, D., Honeyman, M., and J.Jabbal, *Workforce Planning in the NHS*, London, The King's Fund, 2015.

Public health policy and practice: facing the future
David J. Hunter

1   T. Frieden, 'The future of public health', *New England Journal of Medicine*, vol. 373, 2015 pp. 1748-54.

2   D. Wanless, Securing *Our Future Health: taking a long-term view*. London: HM Treasury, 2002.

D. Wanless, *Securing Good Health for the Whole Population*, Final report, London: HM Treasury, 2004.

3   P. Bobbitt, *The Shield of Achilles: war, peace and the course of history*, London: Penguin Books, 2003.

4   B. Butland, S. Jebb, P. Kopelman, K. McPherson, S. Thomas, J. Mardell, and V. Parry, *Tackling Obesities: Future Choices – Project report*, Commissioned by the UK Government's Foresight Programme, Government Office for Science, London: Department of Innovation, Universities and Skills, 2007.

5   R. Dobbs, C. Sawers, F. Thompson, J. Manyika, J. Woetzel, P. Child, S. McKenna and A. Spatharou, *Overcoming Obesity: an initial economic analysis*, New York: McKinsey Global Institute, 2014.

6   NHS England, NHS Five Year Forward View. London: NHS England, 2014.

7   M. Marmot, Fair Society, healthy Lives, The Marmot Review: Strategic Review of Health Inequalities in England post-2010. London: University College London, 2010.

8   D. J. Hunter and L. Marks, 'Health inequalities in England's changing public health system', In: K. Smoth, S. Hill, and C. Bambra, (eds) *Health Inequalities: Critical Perspectives*. Oxford: Oxford University Press, 2015.

9   NHS England, NHS Five Year Forward View, London: NHS England, 2014.

10   A. Tedstone, V. Targett, R. Allen and staff at PHE, *Sugar Reduction: The evidence for action*, London: Public Health England, 2015.

11   J. Popay, M. Whitehead, and D. J. Hunter, 'Justice is killing people on a large scale – but what is to be done about it?', *Journal of Public Health* vol. 32, no. 2, 2010, pp. 150-6.

12   S. Cook, K. Leppo, E. Ollila, S. Pena, and M. Wismar (eds), *Health in All Policies: Seizing Opportunities, implementing Policies*, Helsinki: Ministry of Social Affairs and Health of Finland, 2013.

13   V. Stone, (ed) *Health in All Policies Training Manual*, Geneva: World Health Organisation, 2015.

14   N. Halfon, P. Long, C. Chang, J. Hester, M. Inkelas and A. Rodgers, 'Applying a 3.0 transformation framework to guide large-scale health system reform', *Health Affairs* vol. 33, no. 11, 2014, pp. 2003-11.

15   G. Cooke, and R. Muir (eds.), *The Relational State: how recognising the importance of human relationships could revolutionise the role of the State*, London: Institute for Public Policy Research, 2012.

16   Royal Society for Public Health, *Rethinking the Public Health Workforce*, London: RSPH, 2012.

17   D. Wanless, *Securing Our Future Health: taking a long-term view*, London: HM Treasury, 2002.

Can decentralisation and personal responsibility help re-structure the NHS?

Richard B. Saltman

1   R.B. Fetter, Y. Shin, J.L. Freeman, R.F. Averill, J.D. Thompson, 'Case mix definition by diagnosis-related groups', *Medical Care*, vol. 18 no.2 Suppl. iii 1980, pp. 1-53.

2   S.D. King, *Losing Control: The Emerging Threats to Western Prosperity*, Yale University Press, New Haven and London, 2010.

3   S.D. King, *When the Money Runs Out: The End of Western Affluence*, Yale University Press, New Haven and London, 2013.

4   C. Giles, K. Allen, Southeastern shift: the new leaders of global growth, *Financial Times*, 2013.

5   D. Milliken, A.N. da Costa, 'UK budget deficit widest since 2012 in August after income tax shortfall', Reuters, 22 September 2015.

6   E. Cadman, 'Productivity shortfall stands at widest on record to peers', *Financial Times*, 19 September 2015.

7   J. Wheatley, J. Kynge, 'Emerging markets braced for ripple effect', *Financial Times*, 10 September, 2015.

8   S.D. King, *When the Money Runs Out: The End of Western Affluence*, Yale University Press, New Haven and London, 2013.

9   S. Neville, 'On life support', *Financial Times*, 18 September 2015.

10 R.B. Saltman, Z. Cahn, 'Re-Structuring Health Systems for an Era of Prolonged Austerity', *British Medical Journal: BMJ*, vol. 346 no. f3972 doi: 10.1136/bmj.f3972 (Published 24 June 2013). Print version published 10 August 2013, Vol 347, no. 7920.

11 J. Appleby, *Spending on Health and Social Care over the Next 50 Years: Why Think Long Term?* King's Fund, London, 2013.

12 Mutuals Taskforce, *Public Service Mutuals: The Next Steps.* Cabinet Office, London, 2015.

13 Department of Health, *Examining New Options and Opportunities for Providers of NHS Care: The Dalton Review,* London, December 2014.

14 Five Year Forward View, NHS England, 2014.

15 A. Bounds, 'Manchester's new mayor prepares for 7 billion pound challenge', *Financial Times*, 26 July 2015.

16 R.B. Saltman, V. Bankauskaite, 'Conceptualizing Decentralization in European Health Systems: A Functional Perspective', *Health Economics, Policy and Law*, vol. 1 no. 2, 2006, pp. 127-147.

17 J. Magnussen, K. Vrangback, R.B. Saltman (eds.), *Nordic Health Care Systems: Recent Reforms and Current Policy Challenges,* Open University Press/McGraw-Hill Education, London, 2009.

18 R.B. Saltman, V. Bankauskaite, 'Conceptualizing Decentralization in European Health Systems: A Functional Perspective', *Health Economics, Policy and Law*, vol. 1 no. 2, 2006, pp. 127-147.

19 P. Daneryd, Personal communication, 17 September 2015.

20 R.B. Saltman, V. Bankauskaite, 'Conceptualizing Decentralization in European Health Systems: A Functional Perspective', *Health Economics, Policy and Law*, vol. 1 no. 2, 2006, pp. 127-147.

21 R.B. Saltman, V. Bankauskaite, K. Vrangbaek, (eds.), *Decentralization in Health Care: Strategies and Outcomes.* European Observatory on Health Systems and Policies Series, Open University Press/McGraw-Hill Education, London, 2007.

22 R.B. Saltman, 'Health Sector Solidarity: A Core European Value but with Widely Varying Content', *Israel Journal of Health Policy Research,* 2015, DOI: 10.1186/2045-4015-4-5.

23 H. Schmidt, 'Personal Responsibility for Health: A Proposal for a Nuanced Approach' In: B. Rosen, S. Shortell, A. Israeli (eds.), *Improving Health and Health Care: Who is Responsible? Who is Accountable?*, Israel National Institute for Health Policy Research, Tel Aviv, 2010, pp. 316-344.

24 T. Bodenheimer and K. Lorig, H. Holman, and K. Grumbach, 'Patient Self-management of chronic disease in primary care', *JAMA*, vol. 288 no.19, 2002, pp. 2469-2475, doi:10.1001/jama.288.19.2469.

25 L. Johansson, 'Decentralisation from acute to home care settings in Sweden', *Health Policy*, vol. 41, Supplement S131-144, 1997.

26 N. Genet, W. Boerma, M. Koimann, A. Hutchenson, R.B. Saltman (eds.), *Home Care across Europe: Current Structure and Future Challenges*, vol. I, Occasional Series, European Observatory on Health Systems and Policies, Brussels, 2012.

27 K. Linebaugh, 'Citizen hackers tinker with medical devices', *Wall Street Journal*, 26 September 2014.

28 J. Meikle, 'Minister forces Herceptin U-turn', *The Guardian*, 9 November 2005.

29 S. Boreley, 'Life-extending drugs to be axed by NHS', *The Guardian*, 3 September 2015.

30 S. McIntyre, 'Radiotherapy alternative to be offered in UK after Ashya King's proton therapy "miracle recovery"', *The Independent*, 4 April 2015.

31 T. Hunter, 'Why you WILL have to sell your home to pay for care', *The Telegraph*, 28 February 2015.

32 R. Robinson, 'User charges for health care'. In: E. Mossialos, A. Dixon, J. Figueras, J. Kutzin (eds.), 'Funding for Health Care: Options for Europe', Open University Press, Buckingham, UK, 2002.

33 R.B. Saltman, Z. Cahn, 'Re-Structuring Health Systems for an Era of Prolonged Austerity', *British Medical Journal: BMJ*, vol. 346, no.f3972 doi: 10.1136/bmj.f3972 (Published 24 June 2013). Print version published 10 August 2013, vol. 347, no. 7920.

34 S. Thomson, J. Figueras, T. Evetovits, M. Jowett, P. Mladovsky, A. Maresso, J. Cylus, M. Karanikolos, H. Kluge, *Economic Crisis, Health Systems and Health in Europe*, Open University Press/McGraw-Hill Education, Berkshire, UK, 2015.

35 E. Pavolini, A.M. Guillen, (eds.), *Health Care Systems in Europe under Austerity: Institutional Reforms and Performance*. Palgrave MacMillan, London, 2013.

36 H. Schmidt, 'Personal Responsibility for Health: A Proposal for a Nuanced Approach' In: B. Rosen, S. Shortell, A. Israeli (eds.), *Improving Health and Health Care: Who is Responsible? Who is Accountable?*, Israel National Institute for Health Policy Research, Tel Aviv, 2010, pp. 316-344.

37 H. Schmidt, S. Stock, A. Gerber, 'What can we learn from German health incentive schemes?', *British Medical Journal* vol.339, 2009, pp. 725-728.

38 H. Schmidt, 'Personal Responsibility for Health: A Proposal for a Nuanced Approach' In: B. Rosen, S. Shortell, A. Israeli (eds.), *Improving Health and Health Care: Who is Responsible? Who is Accountable?*, Israel National Institute for Health Policy Research, Tel Aviv, 2010, pp. 316-344.

39 Committee on Choices in Health Care (Dunning Committee), *Strategic choices in health care*, Ministry of Health, Welfare and Sport, The Hague, 1991.

40 G. Tinghogg, P. Carlsson, C.H. Lyttkens, 'Individual Responsibility for What? – A Conceptual Framework for Exploring the Suitability of Private Financing in a Publicly Funded Health-Care System' *Health Economics Policy and Law* vol. 5, no. 2, 2010, pp. 201-224.

41 S. Thomson, J. Figueras, T. Evetovits, M. Jowett, P. Mladovsky, A. Maresso, J. Cylus, M. Karanikolos, H. Kluge, Economic Crisis, Health Systems and Health in Europe, Open University Press/McGraw-Hill Education, Berkshire, UK, 2015.

42 R. B. Saltman, J. Teperi, 'Health Reform in Finland: Current Framework and Unresolved Challenges' (manuscript under review).

43 A. Coulter, *Engaging Patients in Healthcare*, Open University Press/McGraw-Hill Education, Maidenhead, UK, 2011.

44 A. A. Alvarez, and A. Duran, 'Spain', In: R.B. Saltman, A. Duran, and H.F.W. Dubois (eds.), *Governing Public Hospitals,* Observatory Studies Series 25, European Observatory on Health Systems and Policies, Brussels, 2011, pp. 241-260.

The role of predictive technologies in healthcare
Marco Viceconti

1 Auffray, C., Charron, D., and Hood, L. (2010), 'Predictive, preventive, personalized and participatory medicine: back to the future', *Genome Med*, 2 (8), 57.

2 Keller, Evelyn Fox (2003), *Making Sense of Life. Explaining Biological Development with Models, Metaphors, and Machines* (Cambridge, MA: Harvard University Press).

3 El-Metwally, A., *et al.* (2008), 'Genetic and environmental influences on non-specific low back pain in children: a twin study', *Eur Spine J*, 17 (4), 502-8.

4 Katsika, D., *et al.* (2005), 'Genetic and environmental influences on symptomatic gallstone disease: a Swedish study of 43,141 twin pairs', *Hepatology*, 41 (5), 1138-43.

5   Livshits, G., *et al.* (2011), 'Lumbar disc degeneration and genetic factors are the main risk factors for low back pain in women: the UK Twin Spine Study', *Ann Rheum Dis*, 70 (10), 1740-5.

6   Wirdefeldt, K., *et al.* (2011), 'Heritability of Parkinson disease in Swedish twins: a longitudinal study', *Neurobiol Aging*, 32 (10), 1923 e1-8.

7   Obel, N., *et al.* (2010), 'Genetic and environmental influences on risk of death due to infections assessed in Danish twins, 1943-2001', *Am J Epidemiol*, 171 (9), 1007-13.

8   Zdravkovic, S., *et al.* (2002), 'Heritability of death from coronary heart disease: a 36-year follow-up of 20 966 Swedish twins', *J Intern Med*, 252 (3), 247-54.

9   Grossi, E. (2010), 'Artificial Adaptive Systems and predictive medicine: a revolutionary paradigm shift', *Immun Ageing*, 7 Suppl 1, S3.

10   Parikh, N., Zollanvari, A., and Alterovitz, G. (2012), 'An automated bayesian framework for integrative gene expression analysis and predictive medicine', *AMIA Jt Summits Transl Sci Proc*, 2012, 95-104.

11   Smye, S. W. and Clayton, R. H. (2002), 'Mathematical modelling for the new millenium: medicine by numbers', *Med Eng Phys*, 24 (9), 565-74.

12   Taylor, C. A., *et al.* (1999), 'Predictive medicine: computational techniques in therapeutic decision-making', *Comput Aided Surg*, 4 (5), 231-47.

13   Viceconti, M. (2015), 'Biomechanics-based in silico medicine: the manifesto of a new science', *J Biomech*, 48 (2), 193-4.

14   Keller, Evelyn Fox (2003), *Making Sense of Life. Explaining Biological Development with Models, Metaphors, and Machines* (Cambridge, MA: Harvard University Press).

15   Douglas, P. S., *et al.* (2015), 'Clinical outcomes of fractional flow reserve by computed tomographic angiography-guided diagnostic strategies vs. usual care in patients with suspected coronary artery disease: the prospective longitudinal trial of FFRct: outcome and resource impacts study', *Eur Heart J, (in press)*.

16   Morris, P. D., *et al.* (2015), '"Virtual" (Computed) Fractional Flow Reserve: Current Challenges and Limitations', *JACC Cardiovasc Interv*, 8 (8), 1009-17.

17   The interested reader can find a nice overview of how this domain has developed in the various special issues the Royal Society has published over the last few years dedicated to the Virtual Physiological Human, and the recent book edited by

Coveney, Viceconti, and Hunter (Brook *et al.* 2011; P. V. Coveney *et al.* 2013; P. Coveney *et al.* 2014; Gavaghan *et al.* 2009; Kohl *et al.* 2008; Kohl *et al.* 2009; Kohl and Viceconti 2010; Viceconti and Kohl 2010).

18 Pijls, N. H., *et al.* (1996), 'Measurement of fractional flow reserve to assess the functional severity of coronary-artery stenoses', *N Engl J Med*, 334 (26), 1703-8.

19 http://www.heartflow.com

20 Norgaard, B. L., *et al.* (2014), 'Diagnostic performance of noninvasive fractional flow reserve derived from coronary computed tomography angiography in suspected coronary artery disease: the NXT trial (Analysis of Coronary Blood Flow Using CT Angiography: Next Steps)', *J Am Coll Cardiol*, 63 (12), 1145-55.

21 Morris, P. D., *et al.* (2013), 'Virtual fractional flow reserve from coronary angiography: modeling the significance of coronary lesions: results from the VIRTU-1 (VIRTUal Fractional Flow Reserve From Coronary Angiography) study', *JACC Cardiovasc Interv*, 6 (2), 149-57.

22 Lungu, A., *et al.* (2014), 'MRI model-based non-invasive differential diagnosis in pulmonary hypertension', *J Biomech*, 47 (12), 2941-7.

23 Bosi, G. M., *et al.* (2015), 'Patient-specific finite element models to support clinical decisions: A lesson learnt from a case study of percutaneous pulmonary valve implantation', *Catheter Cardiovasc Interv*, (in press).

24 http://feops.com/clinical

25 Gasser, T. C., *et al.* (2014), 'A novel strategy to translate the biomechanical rupture risk of abdominal aortic aneurysms to their equivalent diameter risk: method and retrospective validation', *Eur J Vasc Endovasc Surg*, 47 (3), 288-95.

26 Sforza, D. M., Putman, C. M., and Cebral, J. R. (2012), 'Computational fluid dynamics in brain aneurysms', *Int J Numer Method Biomed Eng*, 28 (6-7), 801-8.

27 Cristofolini, L., *et al.* (2008), 'Multiscale investigation of the functional properties of the human femur', *Philos Trans A Math Phys Eng Sci*, 366 (1879), 3319-41.

28 Falcinelli, Cristina, *et al.* (2014), 'Multiple loading conditions analysis can improve the association between finite element bone strength estimates and proximal femur fractures: A preliminary study in elderly women', *Bone*, 67, 71-80.

29 Qasim, Muhammad, *et al.* (2016), 'Patient-Specific Finite Element Minimum Physiological Strength as Predictor of the

Risk of Hip Fracture: The Effect of Methodological Determinants', *Osteoporosis International* (submitted).

30 Viceconti, M., *et al.* (2008), 'Multiscale modelling of the skeleton for the prediction of the risk of fracture', *Clin Biomech (Bristol, Avon)*, 23 (7), 845-52.

31 Viceconti, M., *et al.* (2012), 'Are spontaneous fractures possible? An example of clinical application for personalised, multiscale neuro-musculo-skeletal modelling', *J Biomech*, 45 (3), 421-6.

32 Bosmans, L., *et al.* (2014), 'Hip contact force in presence of aberrant bone geometry during normal and pathological gait', *J Orthop Res*, 32 (11), 1406-15.

33 Fernandez, J. W., *et al.* (2005), 'A cerebral palsy assessment tool using anatomically based geometries and free-form deformation', *Biomechanics and modeling in mechanobiology*, 4 (1), 39-56.

34 Fregly, B. J. (2009), 'Design of Optimal Treatments for Neuromusculoskeletal Disorders using Patient-Specific Multibody Dynamic Models', *Int J Comput Vis Biomech*, 2 (2), 145-55.

35 Oberhofer, K., *et al.* (2010), 'Subject-specific modelling of lower limb muscles in children with cerebral palsy', *Clin Biomech (Bristol, Avon)*, 25 (1), 88-94.

36 Ravera, E. P., *et al.* (2010), 'Model to estimate hamstrings behavior in cerebral palsy patients: as a pre-surgical clinical diagnosis tool', *Conf Proc IEEE Eng Med Biol Soc*, 2010, 5456-9.

37 Riccio, A. I., *et al.* (2015), 'Three-dimensional computed tomography for determination of femoral anteversion in a cerebral palsy model', *J Pediatr Orthop*, 35 (2), 167-71.

38 Scheys, L., *et al.* (2011b), 'Calculating gait kinematics using MR-based kinematic models', *Gait Posture*, 33 (2), 158-64.

39 Scheys, L., *et al.* (2011a), 'Level of subject-specific detail in musculoskeletal models affects hip moment arm length calculation during gait in pediatric subjects with increased femoral anteversion', *J Biomech*, 44 (7), 1346-53.

40 Weis, J. A., *et al.* (2015), 'Predicting the Response of Breast Cancer to Neoadjuvant Therapy Using a Mechanically Coupled Reaction-Diffusion Model', Cancer Res, (in press).

41 Weis, J. A., *et al.* (2015), 'Predicting the Response of Breast Cancer to Neoadjuvant Therapy Using a Mechanically Coupled Reaction-Diffusion Model', *Cancer Res, (in press)*.

42 Cobelli, C., Renard, E., and Kovatchev, B. (2011), 'Artificial pancreas: past, present, future', *Diabetes*, 60 (11), 2672-82.

43 Britton, O. J., *et al.* (2013), 'Experimentally calibrated population

of models predicts and explains intersubject variability in cardiac cellular electrophysiology', *Proc Natl Acad Sci U S A*, 110 (23), E2098-105.

44 Haddad, Tarek, Himes, Adam, and Campbell, Michael (2014), 'Fracture prediction of cardiac lead medical devices using Bayesian networks', *Reliability Engineering & System Safety*, 123, 145-57.

45 The interested reader can refer to 'In Silico Clinical Trials: How Computer Simulation Will Transform The Biomedical Industry', an international research and development roadmap for an industry-driven initiative that the Avicenna consortium has recently published: http://avicenna-isct.org/roadmap/

46 Carnier, Josh, (2010), 'Siri Personal Assistant: A Voice App That Lets You Speak to OpenTable'. Retrieved from http://blog.opentable.com/2010/siri-personal-assistant-a-voice-app-that-lets-you-speak-to-opentable/>

47 Monegain, Bernie, (2013), 'Health IT outsourcing demands rise'. Retreived from: http://www.healthcareitnews.com/news/health-it-outsourcing-demands-rise